Hospitals

What They Are and How They Work

Third Edition

D0822670

Don Griffin,
FACHE, MS, MBA, JD, LLM

JONES AND BARTLETT PUBLISHERS

Sudbury, Massachusetts

BOSTON   TORONTO   LONDON   SINGAPORE

World Headquarters
Jones and Bartlett
Publishers
40 Tall Pine Drive
Sudbury, MA 01776
978-443-5000
info@jbpub.com
www.jbpub.com

Jones and Bartlett
Publishers Canada
6339 Ormindale Way
Mississauga, Ontario
L5V 1J2
Canada

Jones and Bartlett
Publishers International
Barb House,
Barb Mews
London W6 7PA
United Kingdom

Jones and Bartlett's books and products are available through most bookstores and online book-sellers. To contact Jones and Bartlett Publishers directly, call 800-832-0034, fax 978-443-8000, or visit our website www.jbpub.com.

Substantial discounts on bulk quantities of Jones and Bartlett's publications are available to corporations, professional associations, and other qualified organizations. For details and specific discount information, contact the special sales department at Jones and Bartlett via the above contact information or send an email to specialsales@jbpub.com.

Library of Congress Cataloging-in-Publication Data

Griffin, Don, 1949–
    Hospitals : what they are and how they work / Don Griffin. — 3rd ed.
       p. ; cm.
    Rev. ed. of: Hospitals / I. Donald Snook, Jr. 2nd ed. 1992.
    Includes bibliographical references and index.
    ISBN 0-7637-2758-X (pbk. : alk. paper)
    1. Hospitals. 2. Hospitals—Administration. 3. Hospitals—United States.
  I. Snook, I. Donald. Hospitals. II. Title.
    [DNLM: 1. Hospitals--United States. 2. Hospital Administration
—United States.   WX 100 G851h 2006]
  RA963.S57 2006
  362.11068—dc22

                                2005035985

ISBN-10: 0-7637-2758-X
ISBN-13: 978-0-7637-2758-1
6048

Production Credits
Publisher: Michael Brown
Production Director: Amy Rose
Production Editor: Carolyn F. Rogers
Associate Editor: Kylah Goodfellow McNeill
Associate Marketing Manager:
  Marissa Hederson

Composition: Graphic World
Cover Design: Ryan Wilcox
Cover Image: Photograph used with the
  permission of the University of Michigan
  Health System.
Printing and Binding: Malloy, Inc.
Cover Printing: Malloy, Inc.

Printed in the United States of America
11 10   10 9 8 7 6 5 4 3

Table of Contents

Acknowledgments   xiii
About the Author   xv
Introduction to the Third Edition   xvii

PART I—EVOLUTION OF HOSPITALS   1

Chapter 1—A Brief History   3

   The Very Early Days   3
   Early American Hospitals—From Founding of the
      New World through World War II (1500–1945)   4
   The Modern Era—Post-World War II to the Present
      (1945–2006)   6
   Government Involvement   6
   Summary   7
   Chapter Review   7

Chapter 2—Hospitals and Important Health Care Trends   9

   Types of Hospitals   9
   Important Health Care Trends   9
   Hospital Expenses and Revenues   12
   Summary   16
   Chapter Review   17

PART II—MANAGING THE HOSPITAL **19**

Chapter 3—Organization **21**

Introduction—Common Organizational Management
  Principles 21
How Hospitals Are Organized 22
Line and Staff Functions 23
The Organization Chart 24
A Team of Three—A Very Important Concept 26
Power 26
Corporate Restructuring in the Hospital 26
Multihospital Systems 27
Alliances 27
Chapter Review 27

Chapter 4—The Governing Body **29**

Introduction 29
A Profile of the Governing Body 30
Functions of the Board of Trustees 31
Selection and Evaluation of the Chief Executive Officer .. 33
Relationship with the Medical Staff 33
How Does the Board Operate? 34
Chapter Review 35

Chapter 5—The Chief Executive Officer **37**

Introduction 37
Functions of the Administrator 38
Inside Activities of the CEO 39
Outside Activities of the CEO 40
Assistant Administrator or Vice President 41
The Future for Chief Executive Officers 42
Chapter Review 42

PART III—DOORWAYS TO THE HOSPITAL **43**

Chapter 6—Outpatient Areas **45**

    Introduction   45
    Ambulatory Surgery   46
    Clinics   46
    Ancillary Outpatient Services   47
    Group Practice   47
    Medical Office Buildings (MOBs)   48
    Standards of Accreditation   48
    Major Growth Areas in the Future   49
    Chapter Review   49

Chapter 7—The Emergency Department ....,   **51**

    Introduction   51
    Emergency Department Utilization   52
    Categorization of Emergency Facilities   52
    Physical Facilities   53
    Organization   54
    Admissions   54
    Physician Coverage of the Emergency Department   55
    Records   56
    Financial Implications   57
    Legal Implications   58
    Chapter Review   58

Chapter 8—The Admitting Department **59**

    Introduction   59
    The Department's Role in Public Relations   59
    Functions of the Admitting Department   60
    Types of Admissions   61
    Preadmission   61
    Consent Forms   62
    Bed Assignments   63
    Chapter Review   63

PART IV—THE MEDICAL TEAM **65**

Chapter 9—The Medical Staff **67**

    Introduction 67
    Becoming a Physician 68
    Continuing Medical Education 69
    Organized Medicine 70
    Medical Staff Organization 70
    Closed and Open Medical Staffs 71
    Medical Staff Committees 73
    The Medical Director 74
    The Hospitalist 74
    Allied Health Personnel 74
    Legal Restrictions on Physicians 75
    Chapter Review 75

Chapter 10—Nursing Services **77**

    Introduction 77
    Early Traditions 77
    Nursing Education 78
    Department Organization 80
    The Patient Care Unit 81
    Special Care Units 83
    Modes of Nursing Care Delivery 86
    Terms and Standards 88
    Staffing 88
    Scheduling 89
    Telemonitoring and Bedside Terminals 91
    Nurse Staffing Issues 91
    Chapter Review 92

PART V—TESTS AND RESULTS **93**

Chapter 11—Key Ancillary Services **95**

    Introduction 95
    The Clinical Laboratory Department 96
    The Imaging Department 100

Freestanding Imaging Centers 105
The Anesthesiology Department. 105
Chapter Review 108

Chapter 12—Other Ancillary Services 109

Introduction 109
Respiratory Care Department 109
Electroencephalography 110
The Cardiac Center 111
Rehabilitative Medicine—Physical Therapy, Occupational
Therapy, and Speech Therapy 112
The Pharmacy 113
Chapter Review 117

PART VI—BEHIND THE SCENES—THE SUPPORT SERVICES .. 119
In General, What Are *Support* Services? 119

Chapter 13—Patient Support Services 121

Dietary Department 121
Social Services Department 126
Pastoral Care Services 128
Patient Transportation Services 128
The Patient Representative 129
Chapter Review 129

Chapter 14—Facilities Support Services 131

Introduction 131
Environmental Services Department 131
Hospital Laundry 133
Maintenance Department 134
Plant Engineering. 136
Parking Facilities 136
Security 137
General Safety 137
Fire Safety 139
Disaster Planning 139
Biomedical Engineering 141

Contract Management 142
Chapter Review 143

Chapter 15—Administrative Support Services 145

Introduction 145
Materials Management Department 145
Human Resources Department. 148
The Volunteer Organization 154
Telecommunications Management 155
Chapter Review 155

PART VII—HOSPITAL FINANCES 157

Chapter 16—Generating Revenue 159

Introduction 159
Types of Third-Party Payments 159
The Major Payers 161
Chapter Review 164

Chapter 17—Hospital Budgeting 165

Introduction 165
Types of Budgets 165
Financial and Statistical Reports 166
Chapter Review 169

Chapter 18—Business Functions 171

Introduction 171
The Accountant 172
Hospital Accounting 172
Management Information Systems (MIS) 173
The Public Accounting Firm 174
Patient Accounts and Billing Department 174
Corporate Compliance Programs 175
Chapter Review 175

PART VIII—EVALUATING CARE **177**

Chapter 19—Medical Records **179**

Introduction (HIPAA) 179
Purpose of the Medical Record 180
Manual Medical Records 181
Electronic Medical Records 181
The Medical Records Department 182
Organization of the Department 183
The Medical Records Committee 184
Legal Requirements 185
Medical Records and Quality Improvement 185
Chapter Review 185
Discussion Questions 186

Chapter 20—Quality Improvement **187**

Definition 187
Historical Review 188
Hospital Committees to Advance Quality 189
Chapter Review 192

Chapter 21—Risk Management and Medical Malpractice **193**

Risk Management 193
Risk Management as a Team Approach 193
Risk Management and Quality Improvement 194
Medical Malpractice 194
Defensive Medicine 195
Hospital Liability for Physicians' Acts 195
Respondent Superior 195
Role of the Medical Record 196
Chapter Review 196

Chapter 22—Patient Safety **197**

The Problem of Medical Errors 197
Ending Medical Errors 198
United States vs. European Operating Rooms 199
JCAHO 199
Chapter Review 200

Chapter 23—Bioethics **201**

    Introduction 201
    The Principle of Autonomy 202
    The Principle of Nonmaleficence 203
    The Principle of Beneficence 203
    The Principle of Social Justice 203
    A Final Word 204
    Chapter Review 205
    Discussion Questions 205

Chapter 24—Accreditation and Licensing **207**

    Historical Review 207
    Accreditation Overview 208
    Accreditation in More Detail 209
    What Does Accreditation Really Mean to a Hospital? 210
    Sentinel Events 211
    Joint Commission International 211
    Licensure 211
    Medicare Certification 212
    Registration 212
    Chapter Review 213
    Discussion Question 213

PART IX—CONTINUING TO GROW **215**

Chapter 25—Hospital Marketing **217**

    Introduction 217
    What Is Marketing? 218
    Sales 221
    Branding 222
    Market Research 222
    Market—Studies and Market Audits 222
    Fund-Raising 225
    Chapter Review 225

Chapter 26—Planning **227**

    Introduction 227
    The Evolution of Planning 227
    The Hospital's Long-Range Plan 228
    Who Should Do the Hospital's Planning? 228
    Levels of Long-Range Planning 230
    Benefits of Planning 230
    Planning New Facilities 230
    Chapter Review 231
    Discussion Questions 231

PART X—THE US AND WORLD HEALTH CARE SYSTEMS **233**

Chapter 27—The US Medical Care System **235**

    Introduction 235
    The System's Goals 236
    Outreach Element 237
    Outpatient Element 238
    Inpatient Element 239
    Extended Element 240
    Chapter Review 241

**Chapter 28—The US Health Care System Compared
to the World** **243**

    Introduction 243
    The United States 243
    Cost of Care and Access to Care 244
    Quality of Care 244
    Overseas Opportunities 245
    Chapter Review 245

Appendix A—Case Studies **247**

Appendix B—Glossary **269**

Appendix C—The Hospital: URLs **299**

Index **301**

Acknowledgments

Don Snook, Jr. authored the first two editions of this text, and to his memory, I acknowledge a debt of gratitude. It is my belief that we stand on the shoulders of those who came before us.

I want to acknowledge and thank my father, Richard Griffin, whose career as a hospital administrator set a standard for me to emulate. By observing your experiences and listening to your teachings, I learned an enormous amount . . . thanks, Dad.

To the faculty at Trinity University, especially Dr. Steve Tucker and Dr. Paul Golliher—thank you for providing a solid health care administration education.

To the administrative staff of the Royal Commission Medical Center in Yanbu, Saudi Arabia, especially Mr. Rafat Edrees, Dr. A. El Khider, and Engineer Khalid Radhwan, I owe a large debt . . . you've demonstrated that the fundamentals of health care administration are the same the world over.

Many thanks to Mike Brown and the staff of Jones and Bartlett for having faith in me and allowing me this undertaking.

Finally, the bedrock. Without her kind understanding, prodding, patience, and editorial support, this book would still be between my ears . . . thank you, Polly, my dear wife.

Introduction to
the Third Edition

Medical centers and hospitals are complex businesses offering lifesaving technologies and care to people who are often at their most vulnerable point in life.

This 2006 edition will serve as an up-to-date text for students who wish to build a career in health care, whether as an administrator, nurse, or physician. This text will portray the inner workings of medical centers and hospital organizations by providing the reader with an overview of the governing board, medical staff, and administration. The reader will be guided through the outpatient and emergency departments and then the inpatient areas such ICU, surgery, OB, and various other patient care units. Students will become acquainted with the critical roles played by the different caregivers—the medical staff, nursing, and ancillary members such as laboratory, pharmacy, and imaging personnel. The functions of other departments that support the hospital—dietary, engineering, environmental services, and materials management, to name a few, are described. Transferring to the business side, students will become acquainted with areas of the finance division, such as accounts payable, billing, collecting, and the critical management information systems department. The reader will be introduced to medical records, quality improvement, and risk management—all key elements that work to safeguard patients and the institution.

New features in the third edition include up-to-date descriptions of laws, acts, and regulations affecting health care organizations (HIPAA, etc.). Three new chapters that embrace patient safety issues, current bioethical issues, and how the US health care system and US hospitals compare with those in other countries in the world have been added. Ten case studies portraying problems that administrators sometimes face have also been added; these case studies should provoke lively class discussions.

Part I
Evolution of Hospitals

Chapter 1

A Brief History

THE VERY EARLY DAYS

In the 21st century, it is difficult to imagine that the modern skyscraper medical centers that serve the health care needs of our sprawling communities really started as something quite different. The word *hospital* comes from the Latin word *hospitium*, a word that is mentioned frequently in the literature from the 5th century onward. In early history, *hospitium* meant something quite different from our modern hospital term. A *hospitium* was a place for the reception of strangers and pilgrims.

Following the birth of Christianity, many were encouraged to make pilgrimages to the holy places of the Middle East. For several centuries, travelers from western Europe made their way into this part of the world. These pilgrims traveled without money, believing that they would receive assistance on their route from accommodating citizens.

Many hospitals (in the Greek sense of *hospitium*) were established, particularly in remote and dangerous places. For example, to house pilgrims, it was common for the more well-to-do to bequeath resources to provide the travelers with necessary services. These services were extended as tangible gifts in the spirit of religion. Hospitals were also established by churches as instruments for the propagation of the faith—as living testimonies to their healing missions.

3

Several of the great hospitals can be traced to the period directly following the Council of Nicaea in AD 325, when bishops were instructed to go into every cathedral city to start a hospital. The momentum for the founding of *hospitiums* on the way of the pilgrim was assumed and aided by several knightly orders that took the responsibility of establishing and maintaining these wayside places of rest. The best known of these knightly orders was the Knights of St. John, also known as the Hospitalers.

The oldest operative hospital in the Western world today is probably the Hôtel-Dieu in Paris. This hospital was established around AD 600 by Saint Landry, the Bishop of Paris. Even by current standards, this early French hospital could truly be called a medical center, because it always embraced many of the varied activities necessary to care for the sick.

Though the Crusades gave impetus to the development of hospitals along the road to the Holy Land, travelers returning to England and other parts of western Europe brought back leprosy, which until the time of the Crusades had not been experienced in epidemic proportions in either England or central Europe. About AD 1100, to cope with the spreading leprosy invasion, some 200 hospitals called "lazar houses" were established in England specifically for the care of lepers. This is a large number of hospitals considering that the entire English population at this time was only about three million.

EARLY AMERICAN HOSPITALS—FROM FOUNDING THE NEW WORLD THROUGH WORLD WAR II (1500–1945)

With the exploration of the New World on the North American continent, various French, Spanish, and English colonies were founded. However, none of these settlements brought a lasting system of hospitals. Institutions for the sick, at that time, were simply temporary, makeshift arrangements set up to care for specific illnesses.

Hernando Cortez is credited with establishing the first permanent hospital structure on the North American continent in 1524. The Jesus of Nazareth Hospital is still functioning in Mexico City; it stands as a magnificent example of Spanish architectural genius and a monument to Cortez and the Spanish conquerors of Mexico.

The first hospitals in what is now the United States can be traced to the early 18th century, when continuous service in the form of hospitals was attempted. These were hastily structured arrangements, built primarily to confine contagious diseases during epidemics. They were founded mainly in seaport towns such as New York, Philadelphia, Charleston, South Carolina, and Newport, Rhode Island. These institutions were called almshouses. Established primarily for the urban poor, they were a direct result of urban overcrowding. The first almshouse in the

American colonies was founded in 1713 by William Penn in Philadelphia. It was originally restricted to indigent Quakers, but in 1782 a new building was constructed to serve all the urban poor.

Pennsylvania Hospital in Philadelphia, established in 1751, is considered the oldest voluntary hospital in the United States. Its mission—to serve the sick poor—began to emerge as a result of the efforts of Benjamin Franklin and Dr. Thomas Bond. They championed the cause of Pennsylvania Hospital since little medical attention was provided for the city's poor and mentally ill, while well-to-do residents received medical care in their homes. Pennsylvania Hospital and the hospitals that followed were established in the same general pattern used for such hospitals in England. Pennsylvania Hospital was built with funds appropriated by the provincial legislature and matched by public subscriptions. As patients recuperated, they were required to help pay for lengthy stays by serving food to other patients or by scrubbing floors.

It is important to remember that these early hospitals were devoted generally to the care of the sick, but they were primarily used by the sick homeless and the sick poor. Many physicians did not make use of these hospitals for their private patients. As late as 1908, the Massachusetts General Hospital in Boston still cared only for the poor; physicians were not permitted to charge fees to their patients.

Hospitals also faced an influx of mentally ill patients. The first mental hospital in the current United States was constructed in 1772 in Williamsburg, Virginia, and it carried the descriptive name of Eastern Lunatic Asylum. The humanistic treatment of mental illness within a medical framework was introduced in France by Philippe Pinel in 1796. Pinel's effort was paralleled by Dr. Benjamin Rush in the United States during the same time.

The United States' first Catholic hospital was founded in 1828 by the Daughters of Charity of St. Vincent DePaul in St. Louis. It was called DePaul Hospital. Eight years later, the St. Joseph Infirmary opened in Louisville, Kentucky, as a shelter for orphans and plague victims; it was staffed by the Sisterhood Charity of Nazareth. The reputation of an early American hospital was not enviable. Because the death rate in these hospitals was staggeringly high, due in part to severe epidemics, people considered them a last resort.

Rapidly growing urban centers gave great impetus to the expansion of the American hospital. The need for teaching and research facilities led to the establishment of urban teaching centers and medical school hospitals that continue to be important in training medical students and physicians.

One of the major turning points in the history of hospitals came with the discovery of ether as an anesthetic. The discovery of ether is usually attributed to William T. G. Morton, a Georgia dentist who performed the first hospital surgical procedure using ether in 1846. Crawford Long later reported that he had used ether during an operation in 1842; however, he did not publish reports of his work until after Morton's discovery. The use of ether somewhat reduced the public's fear of hospitals and also accounted for a dramatic increase in surgery.

In the later part of the 19th century, following the work of Louis Pasteur in bacteriology and Joseph Lister in antiseptic surgery, hospitals began to emerge as a place to get well. With the introduction of sulfa drugs in the 1930s and penicillin in the 1940s, it became possible to do surgery with considerably less infection mortality. From that point, hospitals began to acquire a better image for treatment and recovery.

Just as the sick poor spurred the founding of hospitals, the poor also stimulated the origin of organized ambulatory or outpatient care. A Protestant French doctor, Théophraste Renaudot, established free outpatient services for the sick poor in Paris in 1630. In 1641, the drug dispensaries were added. Dispensaries also spread to the New World to serve the urban poor. By the end of the 19th century, there was a decline in the number of dispensaries as hospitals began to develop organized outpatient departments or what we have grown to know as hospital clinics.

THE MODERN ERA—POST-WORLD WAR II TO THE PRESENT (1945–2006)

With the public health movement of the 19th century and the expansion of medical technology following World War II, health threats changed. Acute disease epidemics were replaced by chronic and debilitative diseases. Growing and formidable technology helped to combat some of these illnesses. In 1954, the first successful kidney transplantation took place, and with that, the modern era of transplant medicine began. The technical revolution in human organ transplantation continued with the first heart transplant and the first liver transplant in 1967, the first heart-lung transplant in 1981, and the first permanent artificial heart transplant in 1982. Today, we may be beginning the era of individuals regenerating fresh tissue using their own harvested stem cells.

GOVERNMENT INVOLVEMENT

In the mainstream of medicine's advancing technology, our nation's hospitals are also affected by government involvement and regulation. Since the Commonwealth of Pennsylvania gave the Pennsylvania Hospital a grant in the 1750s, the state and federal governments have provided assistance to our hospitals. In 1948, the Hospital Survey and Construction Act, also known as the Hill-Burton Act, was passed. This legislation provided hospitals—which accepted a commitment to care for the poor—with funds for construction. In 1960, Congress passed the Kerr-Mills bill, which provided joint federal and state assistance for the medically indigent. The largest government involvement occurred in 1965, when the Social Security amendments, Public Laws 89–97, were passed, creating Medicare, a Federal healthcare program for those older than 65 years of age and Medicaid, a program administered by states for the economically challenged. To update Medicare coverage, a recent addition to governmental care was the Medicare Prescription Drug Coverage (effective November 14, 2005), which partially pays for prescription drugs for senior citizens. In 1972, Congress passed additional Social Security amendments, which allowed for the funding of dialysis and transplants for individuals with end-stage renal disease. In 1983, Congress passed legislation targeted toward controlling the ever-increasing costs of the Medicare program by establishing Medicare's diagnostic related groups (DRGs), a prospective payment system (PPS). These, in turn, are evolving into capitated agreements.

Federal legislation such as the Emergency Medical Treatment and Active Labor Act (EMTALA), the Health Insurance Portability and Accountability Act (IIIPAA), and a host of Medicare regulations have affected health care. Following these are more than 50 separate Medicaid plans and, to varying degrees, Certificate of Need (CON) legislation. Health care law has become a new specialty for attorneys.

SUMMARY

Early American hospitals have drawn much of their heritage from European hospitals. However, modern US hospitals have developed rapidly and differently from their early counterparts. Hospitals began to care for the sick almost incidentally. The earliest hospitals were established for pilgrims, the indigent, and plague victims. Later, they became institutions where people from all parts of society could come for diagnosis and recovery.

The hospital, as an institution, has become dynamic in nature; it exists to meet the needs of the people it serves. Today's hospitals continue to make history by reacting to the changing needs of society for better technologies, new services, and greater access.

CHAPTER REVIEW

1. What importance did the Council of Nicaea have in early hospital history?
2. What is the famous Spanish explorer Cortez credited with regarding the history of hospitals?
3. What role did Benjamin Franklin play in early American hospitals?
4. When did physicians begin to transplant organs?
5. What importance did the Hill-Burton Act have?

6. Discuss the difference between Medicare and Medicaid. Why are there so many Medicaid plans?
7. What is a CON? Does your state have such a requirement before large healthcare spending is allowed? Discuss the pros and cons of a CON program.

Chapter 2

Hospitals and Important Health Care Trends

TYPES OF HOSPITALS

Hospitals can be classified in several ways, for example, as a community (acute care) hospital or a non-community hospital (specialty, children's, women's, or perhaps psychiatric), governmental or non-governmental, and for profit or not for profit. They can be classified by bed size—1–74 beds, 75–99 beds, 100–149 beds, etc. Another way is to distinguish rural hospitals from urban hospitals.

In terms of numbers, it is helpful to examine the number of hospitals in several ownership categories (Table 2-1).

In broad terms, it is apparent from the table that nongovernment, not-for-profit hospitals are increasing faster as a percent of total hospitals than the for-profit sector. The number of government hospitals is shrinking at the quickest rate.

IMPORTANT HEALTH CARE TRENDS

Hospital inpatient admissions in the United States have grown from 29,252,000 in 1970 to 33,814,000 in 2001. However, if we make adjustments for the population increase for this same period, we learn that admissions per members

Table 2-1 Number of Community Hospitals by Ownership Type, Various Years

		Nongovernment				Government	
		For profit		Nonprofit			
Year	No. of hospitals	No.	%	No.	%	No.	%
1975	5,875	775	13.2	3,339	56.8	1,761	30.0
1985	5,732	805	14.0	3,349	58.5	1,578	27.5
1995	5,194	752	14.5	3,092	59.5	1,350	26.0
2001	4,908	754	15.4	2,998	61.1	1,156	23.6

Source: *Statistical Abstracts of the United States*, various years; and National Center for Health Statistics (1996).

Table 2-2 Selected Characteristics of Nonfederal, Short-stay Community Hospitals (Various Years 1970–2001)

Measure	1970	1980	1990	2000	2001
No. of hospitals	5,859	5,904	5,420	4,915	4,918
Beds (thousands)	848.2	992.0	929.4	823.6	826.0
Admissions (thousands)	29,252	36,143	31,181	33,089	33,814
Admissions per 1,000 population	144.0	159.6	125.4	117.6	118.7
Resident US population	203.2	226.5	248.7	281.4	284.8
Average length of stay (days)	7.7	7.6	7.2	5.8	5.7
Percent occupancy	78.0	75.4	66.8	63.9	64.5
Outpatient surgeries as a percent of total	-	16.3	50.5	62.7	63.0
Cost per day ($)	74	245	687	1,149	1,217
Cost per stay ($)	605	1,851	4,927	6,649	6,980

Source: *Statistical Abstracts of the United States*, various years; National Center for Health Statistics (1996); and *Health, United States, 2003: With Chartbook on Trends in the Health of Americans*, 2003, Tables 95, 106, and 122.

Table 2-3   Growth in Outpatient Visits for Selected Years

Year	Outpatient visits
1970	133,545,000
2001	539,316,000

Source: AHA Hospital Statistics, 2005 Health Forum LLC.

of the population have actually declined from 144 per thousand to approximately 119 per thousand (Table 2-2).

Instead of being admitted to the hospital, more people than ever are being treated on an outpatient basis. For example, during the period from 1970 to 2001, outpatient visits rose from 133,545,000 to 539,316,000 (Table 2-3). If we divide this by the resident US population, we find outpatient visits per members of the population rose from 0.66 visits per person per year to 1.89 visits per person per year. The number of people admitted is declining by 17%, yet the number of people treated on an outpatient basis has almost tripled. What effect has this had on the hospital industry?

Looking to Table 2-4, we see a continual decline in the number of hospitals, and the number of hospital beds is also lower. The average length of stay (ALOS) is lower as well.

The growth of outpatient procedures and the decline of admissions is perfectly logical. The latest procedures, medications, and imaging devices lead to shorter hospital stays. Many procedures that formerly caused a patient to be hospitalized for several days are now routinely done on an outpatient basis; often the patient is back to work the same week. From 1997 to 2003, the number of ambulatory surgery centers has grown from 2,462 to 3,735 (Figure 2-1).

Table 2-4   Trends in Hospitals, Hospital Beds, and ALOS

Year	Number of hospitals	Number of hospital beds	ALOS
1975	5,979	94,700	7.7
1985	5,784	1,003,000	7.1
1995	5,220	874,000	6.5
2001	4,927	828,000	5.8

Source: AHA Hospital Statistics, 2005 Health Forum LLC.

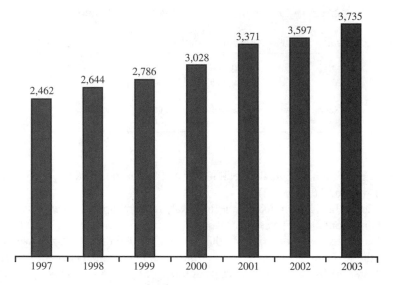

Figure 2-1 Number of ambulatory surgery centers, 1997–2003. *Source:* MedPAC, *Report to Congress*, July 2004.

Rural hospitals have declined during the last 5 years, decreasing from 2,189 in 1999 to 2,166 in 2003 (AHA Hospital Statistics, 2005).

In an effort to survive, hospitals are joining hospital systems and group purchasing organizations. Hospitals reporting they are in a hospital system have increased from 2,524 in 1999 to 2,626 in 2003, and those reporting that they are in a group purchasing organization have increased from 3,080 to 3,650 (AHA Hospital Statistics, 2005).

The number of hospitals has declined. There has also been a decline in the number of beds (though many would argue that in the very recent past, the United States had too many hospitals and hospital beds). On the plus side, the average length of stay has also declined, as have hospital admissions. These are a testament to improvements in medicine, tighter reimbursement systems, and better management.

HOSPITAL EXPENSES AND REVENUES

Hospital revenues and expenses continue to rise each year (Table 2-5).

We can see the percentage of annual hospital expenses growing each year as it is graphed against adjusted admissions (Figure 2-2).

Table 2-5   Hospital Revenues and Expenses Rise Each Year

Year	Total net revenue	Total net expenses
1999	$346.3 billion	$331.22 billion
2000	368.5 billion	353.07 billion
2001	396.1 billion	380.09 billion
2002	431.2 billion	412.52 billion
2003	467.6 billion	445.70 billion

Source: AHA Hospital Statistics, 2005.

Part of the reason for higher expenses is the higher percent change in labor cost of hospital employees versus all service industries (Figure 2-3).

Another reason is the relatively poor rate of reimbursement of the Medicare and Medicaid systems, usually paying below the cost of care (Figure 2-4).

The number of patients who are uninsured also continues to grow (Figure 2-5). Sixty-five percent of uninsured people have full-time jobs but can no longer afford rising health insurance premiums (Figure 2-6).

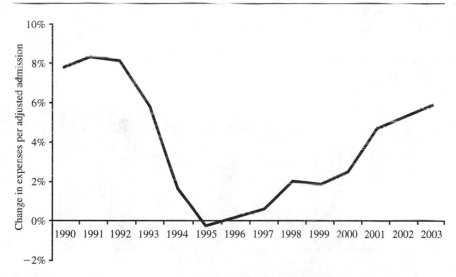

Figure 2-2 Annual change in hospital expenses per adjusted admission, 1990–2003. *Source:* AHA annual survey, 1990–2003. Data is for community hospitals.

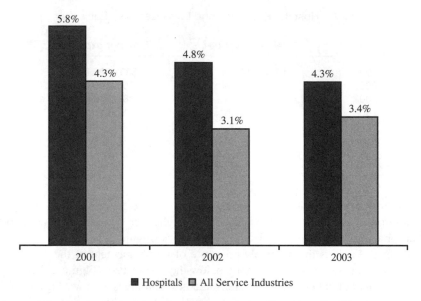

Figure 2-3 Percent change in employment cost index; hospitals versus all service industries, 2001–2003. *Source:* Bureau of Labor Statistics. Data is for total compensation for civilian workers for 12 months ending with the fourth quarter each year.

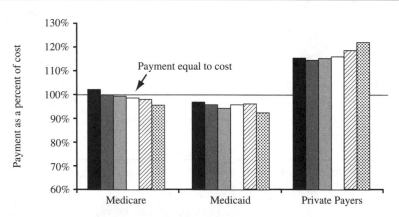

Figure 2-4 Payment relative to cost for Medicare, Medicaid, and private payers, 1998–2003. *Source:* AHA annual survey, 1998–2003. Data is for community hospitals.

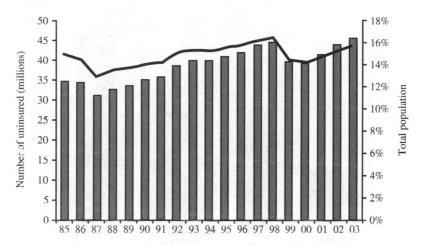

Figure 2-5 Number and percent uninsured, 1985–2003. *Source:* US Census Bureau, *Income, Poverty, and Health Insurance Coverage in the United States: 2003, August 2004.*

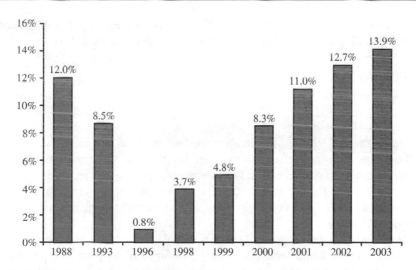

Figure 2-6 Annual percent change in health insurance premiums, 1988, 1993, 1996, 1998–2003. *Source:* The Kaiser Family Foundation and Health Insurance Research and Educational Trust, *Employer Health Benefits*, 1999, 2000, 2001, 2002, 2003.

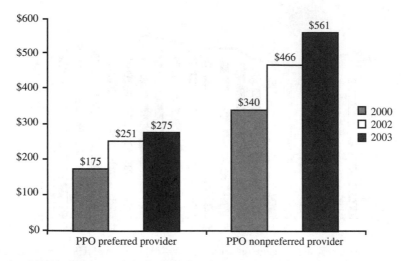

Figure 2-7 Average annual deductible for single coverage in PPO, 2000, 2002, 2003. *Source:* The Kaiser Family Foundation and Health Research and Educational Trust, *Employer Health Benefits*, 2003.

Those with health insurance face a looming problem as their premiums continue to increase at double digit percentages each year (Figure 2-7).

SUMMARY

Hospitals

During the past 30 years, the number of urban and rural hospitals has declined, as have admissions per person. The average length of stay continues to decrease, as does the percent of occupancy. The average cost per day has risen from a mere $74 in 1970 to $1,217 in 2001 and from an average cost per stay of $605 to a tenfold increase of nearly $7,000. This is due, in part, to high labor costs and the high cost of technology.

Hospitals continue to profit from insurance and to break even or lose on Medicare and Medicaid reimbursement. Unfortunately, as insurance premiums rise, the number of people without insurance continues to rise, forcing hospitals to treat many indigent patients.

Outpatient Procedures

The number of outpatient procedures continues to increase dramatically due, in part, to quicker and less invasive medical procedures. The high cost of hospitalization also contributes to the increase.

CHAPTER REVIEW

1. What are five ways that hospitals may be classified?
2. Has the number of hospitals increased or decreased in the United States in the last 30 years? Why?
3. What has caused outpatient visits to increase?
4. What are some reasons for the increased costs of hospital admissions?
5. Why has the average length of stay decreased in hospitals?
6. Why has the number of uninsured people risen in the United States?
7. Discuss the difference in for-profit hospitals and not-for-profit hospitals.
8. Figure 2-4 is the basis for cost shifting. Discuss why.
9. Why have health insurance premiums continued to rise? Discuss important trends.

Part II
Managing the Hospital

Chapter 3

Organization

Key Terms

Alliances	Parent holding company
Bureaucratic organization	Power
Chain of command	Pyramid organization
Classical theory of organization	Span of control
Corporate restructuring	Specialization
Line and staff—the organization chart	A team of three
Multihospital system	

INTRODUCTION—COMMON ORGANIZATIONAL MANAGEMENT PRINCIPLES

One may view a hospital organization with a macro view (such as the Veterans Administration or the Indian Health Service system), or one may consider a micro view and look to departmental organization within the hospital.

Hospitals are mainly bureaucratic organizations and use bureaucratic principles. A principle of bureaucratic organization that applies effectively to hospitals is the grouping of individual positions and clusters of positions into a hierarchy or pyramid.

Another effective principle of hospitals, or, for that matter, any business organization, is the consistent system of rules. Hospital rules are official boundaries for actions within the hospital. Examples of such rules include personnel policies outlined in the personnel handbook and written nursing procedures for patient care in each patient care unit.

Hospitals also use the principle of span of control, which states a manager can effectively supervise only a limited number of people. In a hospital, a span of control of between 5 and 10 people in a given functional area is normal to achieve operational effectiveness. This is especially true in classical functional areas such as housekeeping, dietary, and nursing.

There is also a division and specialization of labor in hospitals. Specialization refers to the ways a hospital organizes to identify specific tasks and assign a job description to each person. For example, a nurse's aide has a specific job that is different from that of a licensed vocational nurse (LVN), sometimes called a licensed practical nurse (LPN), or from that of a registered nurse (RN).

HOW HOSPITALS ARE ORGANIZED

The most popular and traditional hospital structure is a pyramid or hierarchical form of organization. In this arrangement, individuals near the top of the pyramid (e.g., department heads) have a specified range of authority, and this authority is passed down to employees at the lower levels of the pyramid. This is known as a chain of command (Figure 3-1). In this way, hospital authority is dispersed

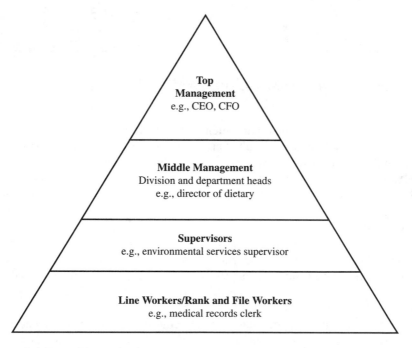

Figure 3-1 Pyramid organization.

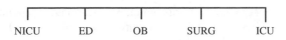

Figure 3-2 Product line management (nursing).

throughout the organization. In hospital pyramid-type structures, supervisors delegate to two or three subordinates who, in turn, delegate down the pyramid.

A second type of organizational scheme is to form teams that are organized for specific projects and for a limited time. An excellent example is preparing for a Joint Commission survey. While the hospital should always be ready when the Joint Commission surveyors arrive, usually an intense effort is begun 12–18 months before the survey is scheduled. Teams can be formed to focus on each standard.

Another example is to form a team to study anticipated projects or product lines before the hospital commits large resources to such an effort. For example, a team could be formed using talented personnel from the accounting, marketing, engineering, and dietary departments to study the cost and profitability of a new food service area, then when the status of the project is decided (go or no go), the team would be disbanded. Teams are a very useful management tool in that they foster cooperation, place authority and responsibility in the hands of those who best know the processes, and can be disbanded easily and reformed for other projects when they arise.

There also could be a hybrid organizational arrangement known as product line management, as shown in Figure 3-2.

Under this scheme, hospitals or divisions within hospitals are organized according to product line categories. These categories may be referred to as strategic business units. For example, a hospital might elect to organize around its surgical or obstetrical services (called products), within formal departments such as nursing.

LINE AND STAFF FUNCTIONS

Another important principle of organization that works well in the hospital is the differentiation between line and staff work. Perhaps the best way to view the difference between line and staff is to regard the line authority in the hospital as advocating direct supervision over subordinates (e.g., the nurse manager is directly responsible for the work of employees under the nurse manager's supervision). The delineation between line and staff is very noticeable in the nursing services department; managers (that is, directors, assistant directors, supervisors, and nurse managers) carry out the line authority, and the educational component (in-service nursing) is an advisory or staff function that supports the line authority.

THE ORGANIZATION CHART

The governing body of the organization is generally referred to as the board of governors, board of trustees, or board of directors. The board hires the chief executive officer (CEO), who may have the title of director, administrator, or president of the hospital; the board assigns authority to that person. The CEO usually has some flexibility in structuring the administration of the hospital, as shown in the lower half of the organization chart (Figure 3-3). But the same general administrative hierarchical principles apply. Depending on the size of the organization, the administrator generally has associate administrators, assistant administrators, or administrative assistants to handle various organizational and operational aspects of the day-to-day functioning of the hospital. It is usual for a CEO to have support from a vice president, chief operating officer (COO), or other assistant administrators. The number of such executive vice presidents will vary by hospital size. It is common for hospitals in the 200–300 bed range to have three or four assistant administrators. Generally, this number will increase proportionately to the number of beds in the hospital. The organization chart illustrates how the span of control for the CEO and the vice presidents follows the span of control principle in the classical organization theory. In a small hospital (100 beds), there may be three vice presidents—one for finance, one for nursing, and one for ancillary and support services. In larger hospitals, vice presidents may have fewer departments.

Secondary to the vice president level in the hospital organization chart is the middle management group. This represents the departmental level of management. In the departmental or functional organization of the hospital, there are generally four major types of functions to be carried out: 1) nursing functions, 2) business or fiscal functions, 3) ancillary or professional services, and 4) support services. It is usual in a hospital to have at least four distinctive administrative or functional groupings answering to the CEO with a vice president responsible for each of the areas. Frequently, CEOs and managers portray their organization charts as was done in Figure 3-3.

Although an organization chart serves a purpose, in many instances it also has severe limitations. One of the limitations is that it does not show the hospital's informal organization. In addition, physicians and other members of the medical staff generally do not appear in any formal authority relationships on most organization charts. Although many resources of the hospital are often available to the physician in order to meet the physicians' and the patients' needs, hospitals have not been able to show effectively the resulting relationships on most organizational charts.

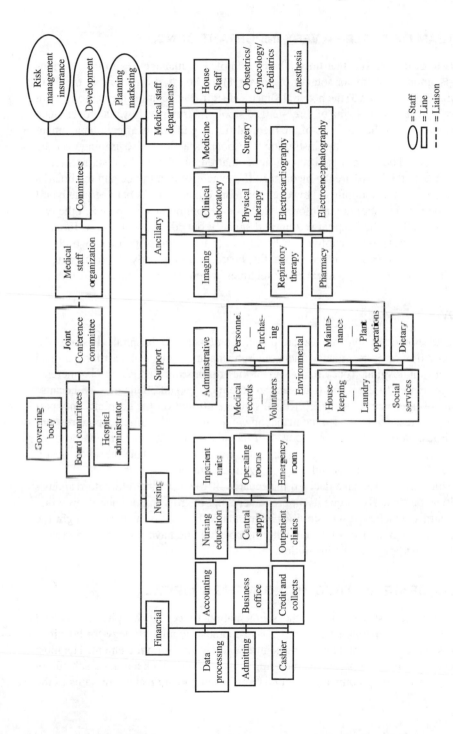

Figure 3-3 A typical hospital organization chart.

A TEAM OF THREE—A VERY IMPORTANT CONCEPT

One of the reasons that hospitals are complex to manage lies in the relationships among three major sources of power: 1) the board of directors, 2) the CEO or management, and 3) the hospital's medical staff. The relationships among them may be regarded as a kind of three-legged stool or a tripartite hospital governance concept. Just as the activities of the medical staff significantly affect management and the governance of the institution, the board's actions also impinge on the physicians. The main organizational units that enable the medical staff to relate formally to the board are the medical staff's executive committee and the board's joint conference committee. However, the more dynamic links between the board and the medical staff are in informal day-to-day communication between the two groups, both in the hospital setting and socially outside the institution. In addition, many hospitals have found it beneficial to have one or perhaps two physicians serve as voting members on the board. Consequently, there is a team approach to hospital organization, sometimes called a team of three.

POWER

One should not generalize about power relationships in hospitals. Historically, the board of directors, management, and physicians or medical staff have all had power in a hospital. Today the power of the administrator appears to be increasing compared to the board (trustees) and the medical staff. This may be because many of the physicians on the medical staff are present (in the hospital) only part time, whereas the CEO and the management team have full-time hospital responsibilities. Despite the growing power of the administrator, there are more physicians employed in and using hospitals than ever before. Their presence is still integral to both hospitals and the organization of those hospitals.

Since US courts have decided that boards of trustees have ultimate responsibilities, particularly in quality improvement, the board's importance is growing. A board's fiduciary responsibilities as mandated by the courts have brought the trustees into greater involvement with the hospital and have given them a greater stake in the power of the institution.

CORPORATE RESTRUCTURING IN THE HOSPITAL

Corporate restructuring, or the segmentation of certain hospital assets and functions into separate corporations, has become a popular strategy for hospitals to assist them in adapting to changes in regulations and reimbursement. The most common form of corporate restructuring is when a hospital becomes a subsidiary of a parent holding company or foundation. Inpatient care usually remains as the primary function of the hospital corporation, and nonprovider functions may be transferred to other corporations related to the hospital. The parent holding company and nonhospital subsidiaries are able to enter into less restrictive joint ventures with physician groups and other health care providers than would be allowed by the traditional hospital structure. The traditional reasons for corporate restructuring include the optimization of third-party reimbursement, tax considerations, government regulation, flexibility, and diversification.

MULTIHOSPITAL SYSTEMS

An increasing number of freestanding hospitals are becoming part of a larger multihospital system. A multihospital system is two or more hospitals that are managed, leased, or owned by a single institution. Some of the common advantages of multihospital systems include economies of scale with management and purchasing, the ability to provide a wide spectrum of care, and increased access to capital markets.

ALLIANCES

Another development among nonprofit hospitals has been the creation of alliances. An alliance is a formal arrangement among several hospitals and/or hospital systems that establishes written rules for its members to follow. Unlike hospitals within a multihospital system, those in an alliance retain their autonomy. The advantage of an alliance is the development of a network of support among hospitals. For example, hospitals might join in an alliance to gain purchasing power or form a preferred provider organization to offer selected services to customers or patients at special rates. A disadvantage is that antitrust issues may arise from such alliances; each hospital's legal counsel should be consulted before the hospital commits to an alliance.

CHAPTER REVIEW

1. What is a chain of command?
2. Discuss the difference between line and staff functions.
3. What is span of control?
4. What is product line management?
5. What are some advantages of forming teams to undertake work and projects? Disadvantages?
6. Discuss the concept of corporate restructuring. What are the pros and cons for a hospital?

7. You are the CEO of a 200-bed free-standing hospital in a large city with 36 other hospitals. Discuss the pros and cons of becoming part of a multi-hospital system.

8. Review question 7, but instead of becoming part of the multihospital system, you consider joining an alliance. What are the pros and cons?

Chapter 4

The Governing Body

INTRODUCTION

In a not-for-profit hospital the governing body, which is also referred to as the board of trustees, board of directors, or board of governors, is the organized entity that bears the ultimate responsibility for all decisions that are made within the hospital. The board essentially functions as the owner of the hospital and is accountable to the community. Board members are often elected by the community just as school board members are elected. They hire and terminate the CEO/administrator.

This concept differs in for-profit companies that own many hospitals. While the for-profit company has a corporate board at their central headquarters, each of their individual hospitals within the company may have its own local governing board, whose members are usually appointed by the local administrator (who is an employee of the for-profit company). This second board generally gives advice to help safeguard the community's best interests. This local board can only make recommendations (and can recommend to the company that the administrator be replaced, since he/she is an employee of the company and not the local hospital—often the for-profit company will replace a valued administrator by simply transferring them to a different company hospital).

Trustees undertake the ultimate responsibilities of managing the hospital's assets and of setting policy; they assume a fiduciary responsibility (defined as a

29

"greater than normal duty"—this concept is seen between attorneys and their clients or physicians and their patients). The courts have found that the governing body is responsible for all activities within the hospital. Members who serve on the governing body clearly have a significant responsibility.

Trustees are private citizens who often want to help their neighbors and community. One of the original reasons for selecting private citizens as hospital trustees was to secure financial support for the institution. By appointing local citizens who had some influence and affluence, the hospital could guarantee a certain amount of contributions to underwrite the care of the poor and the hospital's overall operation. In years past, hospital boards were often appointed so that the hospitals could obtain monetary benefits from their members; now hospital boards frequently appoint individuals who have particular skills that can help the hospital, e.g., with legal advice, accounting assistance, or business and management support. Today's hospital has a multitude of legal and accreditation requirements. The board of trustees is required by law to watch over the hospital and its operations.

Nonprofit hospital trustees generally serve without pay; they are prohibited from profiting financially from their membership on the board of trustees. The rewards for being a trustee are the satisfaction of having delivered a service to others in the community and the acceptance of some measure of community status by being on the board. However, they have the additional burden of protecting the patients from all foreseeable and preventable harm—they accomplish by approving each medical staff member.

In part because of the scandals at Enron, Tyco, and other corporations, there has been an increased sensitivity to board oversight and to conflicts of interest in our American institutions. As part of a public service establishment, hospital trustees may be vulnerable to lawsuits and should check that the hospital carries director and officer (D&O) insurance on their behalf.

Hospitals are increasingly coming under public scrutiny. Some areas, including New York City and Washington, DC, have prohibited hospital trustees from doing business directly or indirectly with the hospitals in which they serve. More commonly, a state will require that trustees make full public disclosure of their business interests and dealings with the hospital that they represent. Hospitals are well advised to comply fully with procedures for disclosing conflicts of interest, even though it can be shown in many cases that overlapping trustee interests can actually work to the hospital's benefit. For example, a trustee might give an institution a favorable loan or expert advice on investments.

A PROFILE OF THE GOVERNING BODY

Just as hospitals vary considerably in size, purpose, and makeup, so do their boards. The average hospital board today has 17 members. The smaller boards may have 8 or 9 members and the larger boards have around 25 members.

Typically, a board is predominately composed of business executives, but it may include members of the legal and accounting professions. Physicians sometimes serve as representatives of the medical staff but may or may not have voting power. Interest and commitment to the hospital, followed by financial business skills are the leading criteria for selecting trustees. Trustees are frequently chosen from among the more outstanding members of the community. It is common to find representatives with inherited wealth serving on boards. A more recent trend, however, has been one of providing community or consumer representation on boards. Yet, for the most part, the traditional character of the board still holds. As to the age of a typical board member, we can generalize that about half are older than 50. The majority of board members have a business or health care background. The majority of hospitals have their own CEO as a board member, but usually only a small percentage grant the CEO voting privileges.

Potential trustee qualifications must be carefully reviewed. Hospital trustee-ship demands certain essential traits, including dedication to hospital business, management skills, involvement in the community, political influence in the community, and a cooperative attitude.

As mentioned in the chapter introduction, in some areas of the country, hospital boards are similar to school boards in that board members are elected by the local citizenry. In these rural areas and small towns, it is common to have an election every 2 years and elect a portion of the board. Civic-minded people usually run for the board but often these people are not the most informed in hospital matters. An additional caveat is that each board member may see themselves as the boss of the CEO, instead of collectively acting with one voice. Horror stories abound among rural administrators, including tales of individual board members wandering the halls of the hospital, attempting to order employees to do certain tasks. It is the wise CEO who brings in an outside consultant for periodic board member education, instilling a *collective spirit* within the board so they act with one voice and stay within their agreed bounds of distant oversight.

Hospital boards typically meet from 10 to 12 times a year, usually on a monthly basis. This is reasonable considering a board might not meet during one of the summer months or during the holiday season. Board terms vary considerably, but the average term of membership is slightly in excess of 3 years with a majority of hospitals stipulating no limit on the number of consecutive terms a board member may serve.

FUNCTIONS OF THE BOARD OF TRUSTEES

The basic function of the governing body is to protect and guide the hospital's mission in accordance with the institution's structure and the needs of the community. Since the board of trustees has an explicit or implicit obligation to act on behalf of the community's interest, it has a fiduciary responsibility to the

community. This responsibility is founded upon trust and confidence. It involves:
1) the formal and legal responsibility for controlling the hospital and assuring the
community that the hospital works properly, 2) overseeing that the hospital acts
in a fiscally responsible manner, 3) appointing and removing members of the
medical staff, and 4) appointing a capable chief executive officer.

Hospital trustees help to set hospital policies. These policies are general written statements or understandings that guide or channel the thinking and action of
the medical staff and the administrator in decision making. The trustees' functions are summarized in Exhibit 4-1.

Exhibit 4-1 Primary functions of the board of trustees.

Members of a board of directors or a board of trustees attain their positions in one of three
ways. They are either elected by their fellow citizens (such as school board members or hospital district board members), are appointed by county officials (such as the county judge
appointing county hospital board members), or are appointed by company officials, in the case
of for-profit hospital companies appointing local citizens to their local hospital board. Most
boards usually derive their authority and power from the hospital charter that created the hospital, or from state statutory regulations.

To encapsulate major points of the board's functions, it is nearly universally agreed that
boards serve to:

- Interview, appoint, and sometimes discharge the chief executive officer.
- Engage in periodic strategic planning with the CEO and key medical and senior hospital staff members.
- Provide a mission statement that meets the needs of the hospital's target population. In
  this regard, the board should periodically discuss with the CEO his/her vision for the
  future and the board should assist in goal setting.
- Assist in providing a sound financial platform—this can be, but is certainly not limited
  to, a monthly review of key financial statements, a review of the annual budget, approval
  of spending for major capital equipment, approval of all hospital contracts, and approval
  of all insurance products.
- Approve of all additions to and changes in the medical staff. The board also reviews and
  approves all changes to medical staff bylaws and standards. The Joint Commission on
  Accreditation of Healthcare Organizations (JCAHO) carefully reviews this aspect to
  insure the board is appropriately carrying out its oversight function.
- Be a liaison with the public to assist the public's understanding of the mission of hospital. Board members may be popular speakers for civic organizations and should represent the hospital when necessary.

Boards are often regulated by local, county or state regulations. Members must be thor-
oughly familiar with open meeting laws and statutes that address conflict of interest issues.
Wise hospital boards should insure coverage through director and officer insurance policies.
As the guiding hand, board members are liable for potential litigation.

In a hospital system there may be a local board of trustees and a corporate board of the multihospital system. However, the local governing body retains primary responsibility for key medical staff relationships. The assumption of a role as a trustee in a multihospital system need not mean the loss of autonomy of the local hospital governing board.

SELECTION AND EVALUATION OF THE CHIEF EXECUTIVE OFFICER

To assist the board of trustees in managing the hospital, the trustees have an obligation to hire a competent chief executive officer to oversee the day-to-day management of the hospital. One of the board's most important functions is the investigation, review, and selection of the CEO. Hospitals are a big business, and trustees must seek executives who have strengths in planning, organizing, and controlling, as well as proven leadership skills. The board then delegates to the CEO the authority and responsibility to manage the everyday operations of the hospital while retaining the ultimate responsibility for everything that happens in the hospital. The relationship between the CEO and the governing board is primarily that of employee-employer, but not in the usual sense of the term. Since the hospital is a very special type of organization, the relationship between the CEO and the governing board is in fact similar to a partnership. Just as it is the responsibility of the governing board to hire the CEO, it is also their responsibility to discharge the CEO if necessary. Determining if this is necessary can best be accomplished by having a contractual arrangement described in clearly understandable terms.

RELATIONSHIP WITH THE MEDICAL STAFF

The hospital medical staff operates under its own bylaws, rules, and regulations, but the physicians on the medical staff are accountable to the board of trustees for professional care of their patients. The board of trustees is responsible for exercising care in the appointment of physicians to the staff. The medical staff carefully reviews a physician's application file, including credentials and privileges requested. The medical staff then recommends to the board of trustees which privileges should be granted to the applicant. The trustees act upon these recommendations. The board could choose to grant privileges, to request further information from the medical staff, or to reject privileges outright.

The board of trustees is legally responsible for care provided in the hospital by attending physicians and hospital employees. The courts pointed out in *Darling v. Charleston Community Memorial Hospital* that the board of trustees has a duty that may go beyond simple delegation of authority to the medical staff. In the Darling case, the court held that the hospital corporation was liable because it did not intervene through its employees to prevent damage that occurred to a patient through the negligence of one of the hospital's physicians. In another landmark case in 1973, the courts found in the case of *Gonzales v. John J. Nork, MD, and Mercy General Hospital of Sacramento, California*, that a hospital owes the patient a duty of care. In this case, Dr. Nork performed 36 unnecessary operations over a 9-year period. The court noted that the board of trustees has an obligation to purge the hospital of incompetent physicians. This case reconfirmed the board's corporate responsibility for quality. It cannot be delegated.

The CEO and the chief/president of the medical staff also have major roles to play. Together with the board, they develop and implement a quality improvement program. The board's job is to monitor the program. This includes receiving monthly reports on the medical staff's performance as measured against standards, concurring with medical staff recommendations, or developing the board's own recommendations to improve quality in the institution.

Boards of trustees generally delegate the daily hospital medical affairs to the medical staff. The medical staff carries out these functions according to its own bylaws and regulations, but these bylaws and regulations are periodically re viewed and approved by the board. The board's joint conference committee has representatives from the medical staff and administration and serves as the main committee between the medical staff of the board and its administrator.

HOW DOES THE BOARD OPERATE?

The board of trustees operates under the bylaws of the hospital. The bylaws spell out how a hospital board operates to attain its objectives. Typical bylaws include a statement on the hospital's purpose and the responsibilities of the board. They also contain a statement of authority for the board to appoint the administrator and the medical staff. Additionally, bylaws outline how board members are appointed and for what period. Most bylaws indicate an elaborate committee structure. It is through these board of trustees committees that the governing board usually accomplishes its goals. This committee structure is frequently established along special functional lines. There is remarkable consistency throughout the nation's hospitals in board committee structure. Perhaps the reason for this consistency is the impetus toward review of hospital bylaws and suggestions from the JCAHO.

The most common committee is the executive committee, which exists in the vast majority of hospitals. Other examples could include a finance committee and a planning committee. Generally, recommendations through the separate committees affect the governance, management, and administration of the hospital, as well as the hospital's medical staff.

It is the duty of the board to carefully select the members of these board committees. The caliber of the recommendations that emerge from these committees and subsequently the caliber of the resulting board action is frequently a result of the quality of the committee assignments. Through the application of leadership skills and management delegation and in close relationship with these board committees, the CEO frequently provides the ultimate key to success in all aspects of the hospital operation.

Hospital boards are operating more and more like other corporate boards. Corporate board members are accustomed to providing an independent voice. Clearly, hospital trustees are respected for their independence and their overview of the hospital. This is the result of an increasing need to make hospitals more efficient and competitive.

CHAPTER REVIEW

1. What is meant by *fiduciary*?
2. How do not-for-profit and for-profit boards differ?
3. Why is director and officer insurance important?
4. What are five functions of the board of directors?
5. What is the importance of the board's bylaws?
6. Discuss the profile of a typical hospital board member. How might have the person become a member of the board?
7. What relationship does the board of directors have with the medical staff? Discuss at least three important things the board does that directly affect the hospital's physicians.

Chapter 5

The Chief Executive Officer

Key Terms	
American College of Health Care Executives (ACHE)	Inside activities
	Networking
Chief executive officer (CEO)	Outside activities
Chief operating officer (COO)	*Respondent superior*
Ex officio member	

INTRODUCTION

Chief executive officers (CEOs), also referred to as hospital administrators, come from many backgrounds. At one time, it was likely that they were chosen from the ranks of the nursing department. In many religion-based hospitals, it was common for the CEO to be selected from the ranks of the religious order or from among retired clergy. On the other hand, some administrators worked their way up through the business office ranks to become the hospital's CEO. It was also common in some hospitals to have a retired executive or physician assume the CEO position.

Such upward, vertical mobility is not common today. CEOs are now products of universities. The first university course for hospital administrators started in the mid-1930s. As the field of hospital administration became more and more complex following World War II, the demand for trained hospital administrators multiplied. One of the greatest influences on the advancement of hospital administration was the formation of the American College of Health Care Executives (ACHE) in 1933. The college encourages high standards of education and ethics, and only those administrators who meet the college's requirements are admitted as members. Today, a number of universities in the United States and Canada provide formal training of hospital administrators. These universities offer graduate and undergraduate degrees in hospital or health care administration.

The master's degree (required for the CEO in most hospitals) is most widely accepted as the academic preparation for health administration; usually this is a master of science in health care administration (MS-HA). Many choose instead a master of business administration (MBA), although some pursue a master of public administration (MPA) or a master of public health (MPH) degree. The formal training program for hospital administrators covers three general areas: 1) administrative and business theory, 2) the study of various components of health care services and medical care, and 3) the study of hospital functions, including the organization and management within the hospital and the role of the hospital in the larger picture of health care delivery systems. The three basic types of skills developed in training are technical, social, and conceptual.

FUNCTIONS OF THE ADMINISTRATOR

The hospital CEO of the 1930s and 1940s chiefly conducted inside activities, that is, he or she dealt primarily with internal operations of the hospital. The administrator was concerned with matters that directly affected patients treated at the hospital. This involved bargaining with employees, developing proper benefit packages, and determining the best methods and techniques to manage the institution. However, beginning in the 1950s and continuing into 1970s, increasingly strong labor unions, third-party payers, and governmental agencies all began to significantly affect the hospital industry. During this period, the role of the administrator became a dual one, dealing with issues both inside the hospital and those that are outside, or external. More sophisticated and specialized management was required to operate a hospital effectively, and the CEO became more involved in activities outside the hospital.

Today the CEO has to strike the proper balance between outside and inside activities. It is typical today for the CEO to delegate the everyday hospital operations to the assistant administrator/chief operating officer (COO), who is often also in charge of all of the ancillary and support services departments. The CEO might spend about 80% of his or her time outside the hospital visiting members of the medical staff in their offices or visiting members of the board or officials of local government.

According to the ACHE, the governing authority appoints a chief executive who is responsible for the performance of all functions of the institution and is accountable to the governing authority. The chief executive, as the head of the organization, is responsible for all functions, including the medical staff, nursing division, patient support services, technical support, and general services support, which will be necessary to assure the quality of patient care. In many cases, the CEO also leads in recruiting new members of the medical staff.

INSIDE ACTIVITIES OF THE CEO

Inside activities include duties such as the review and establishment of hospital procedures, supervision of hospital employees, and operations that include fiscal activities and the maintenance of internal relations. Traditionally, the CEO's job is to attend to those tasks that directly affect patients. For example, it is the responsibility of the CEO to see that the building and its facilities are in adequate order and that personnel are qualified to fill their specific job requirements. Legally, the CEO must answer for acts of employees under the principle of *respondent superior* (a Latin phrase meaning the master is responsible for the acts of the servant). Another traditional CEO function, which is even more important today, is to deal with the hospital's physicians. The administrator must keep both the physicians and the governing board informed about the hospital and its plans. Other important tasks involve recruitment of new medical staff and retention of existing staff.

Generally, CEOs attend board meetings in order to communicate ideas, thoughts, and policies that will aid the hospital. The CEO assigns the responsibility to prepare annual budgets to the chief financial officer, the director of nurses, and the assistant administrator. The budgets will then be presented by the CEO and be approved or changed by the board of trustees. This process includes identifying services that need to be offered as well as equipment that needs to be purchased. While the CFO usually negotiates reimbursement rates with third-party insurance plans (such as Blue Cross and Medicare) and prepares monthly financial statements and statistical data to present to the board, the CEO should always review these documents with the CFO before they are presented to the board.

Maintaining a positive relationship and effective communication with the hospital's governing body, medical staff, employees, and patients is important. The official relationship between the CEO and governing body is that of an employer and employee but actually the CEO and the board function more as partners. The administrator is the representative of the board in the institution's daily activities and must turn the board's power into administrative action. When administrators are members of the board they have the title of president of the institution and report to the chairman of the board. CEOs can become active with voting privileges or act as ex officio members on strategic board committees, including nominating, bylaws, and planning committees. However, it is not common for the CEO to be chairman of the board.

The CEO should act in partnership not only with the board of trustees but also with physicians and with other health care personnel in the institution. Under the best circumstances, the administrator has a mutual understanding with, respect for, and trust in members of the medical staff. One of the key responsibilities of the chief executive officer is to communicate with the hospital's medical staff. It is the CEO's job to see that the physicians have the proper tools in the right place at the right time in order to carry out their roles in the hospital.

Successful CEOs must be effective in keeping their medical staff members informed about organizational changes, board policies, and decisions that affect them and their patients. Hospital medical staffs, though ultimately answerable to the board and its management, are also self-governing and have their own bylaws. The administrator should be sensitive to the medical staff's needs for self-governance and support. From time to time, natural tensions will arise between the medical staff and the administration. Frequently the sources of this conflict can be attributed to poor communication. The CEO must communicate effectively with the medical staff if the hospital is to function efficiently. Consequently, the CEO must always be available to medical personnel. It is a good idea for the CEO to attend the monthly medical staff meeting in order to foster good communications.

The employee group provides many of the CEO's day-to-day challenges. Employees must look to the CEO as their work leader. In this capacity, the CEO must keep employees informed of the critical role their services play in the successful operation of the hospital. This is easier to achieve with nurses and others who deliver direct patient care, but the CEO must continually inform all employees of their mission and importance. While managing employees at all levels, it is critical that the CEO show objectivity, understanding, and fairness. The CEO must exercise the authority to employ, direct, discipline, and dismiss employees with these important principles in mind.

Finally, the CEO has a vital role in patient relations. The CEO must fulfill all legitimate patient requests for general comfort and care in order to assist patient recovery. In dealing with patients, the CEO must also understand the needs of the patients' friends and relatives. It is important that the CEO insure that confidential patient information is protected.

OUTSIDE ACTIVITIES OF THE CEO

Outside activities of today's CEOs are numerous. They include periodically visiting all physicians in the community and encouraging their use of the hospital, relating information to the community about the hospital, building relationships with and lobbying government contacts, and participating in educational and planning activities. One of the roles of the modern administrator is to educate the community about hospital operations and health care matters. This is usually done through hospital publications and community lectures. It is the CEO's responsibility to present a positive image of the hospital. Public relations duties are considered key outside activities, and the CEO must promote public understanding of hospital programs through the mass media.

One of the most valuable accomplishments of today's CEO is the negotiating of contracts with third-party payers (insurance companies) who pay the patients' bills. This is a time-consuming activity requiring a combination of management and negotiation skills. With the advent of Medicare in 1966, hospitals and government became more deeply intertwined. Today's CEO must stay on top of the latest government rules and regulations concerning funding, reimbursement, and planning issues. CEOs meet with governmental reimbursement agencies, planning bodies, and politicians in order to stay current and to lobby for hospital interests. CEOs may lobby on an individual basis, with area CEOs, or as part of regional or national groups through hospital associations.

Interacting with public vendors and other health administrators and agencies is vital to the CEO's mission. The CEO's job is to remain in close contact with the community that sponsors the hospital or health care institution. The CEO must realize that the institution has a responsibility to the public and that the public has a right to be informed. The CEO has to maintain high ethical principles in dealing with vendors. The CEO must maintain impartiality and objectivity when representing the hospital in business transactions. Neither the institution nor the administrator can accept favors, commissions, unethical rebates, or gifts from vendors in turn for doing business with a certain company.

Frequently, CEOs telephone each other or meet to gain additional information on a particular topic, insight, or problem, or just to discuss institutional plans and situations. This professional courtesy helps administrators to broaden their own perspectives and strengthen their problem-solving abilities. This is referred to as networking. However, discussing pricing or agreeing to which hospital will deliver which services is probably counterproductive—and possibly also in violation of antitrust laws.

ASSISTANT ADMINISTRATOR OR VICE PRESIDENT

One of the most important responsibilities of the CEO is to select and hire a competent administrative staff. The administrator's staff is given the responsibility of seeing that the hospital is run smoothly and efficiently. The assistant administrator or vice president, sometimes referred to as the chief operating officer (COO), is in charge of hospital operations and assists the CEO in coordinating all hospital activities such as support, ancillary, and fiscal services. Typically, there are assistant administrators or vice presidents in charge of all major functional areas in the hospital.

The administrative assistant is frequently involved in staff functions and is a junior member of the hospital's administrative team. The administrative assistant plans and participates in studies and programs that help the CEO in the hospital.

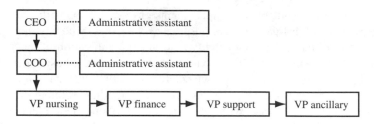

Figure 5-1 Typical organization of vice presidents.

Frequently the administrative assistant is a liaison between the hospital administrator and some of the other functioning hospital departments.

THE FUTURE FOR CHIEF EXECUTIVE OFFICERS

Although hospitals are not growing in numbers, they certainly have become much more complex, and by doing so, they have created a middle management level, which means more management positions for health care administrators. Other changes in the health care industry are also creating new jobs in hospital administration such as VP of Regulatory Affairs and VP of Corporate Compliance. With respect to female hospital administrators, the future looks bright. A review of the number of students who are entering graduate programs in hospital administration shows nearly an equal number of men and women.

CHAPTER REVIEW

1. What are some functions of the CEO?
2. What do we mean by activities outside the hospital?
3. What are some activities inside the hospital that should concern the CEO?
4. What is the typical function of the COO?
5. Discuss the term *respondent superior*. If an employee is sent to a local hardware store for plumbing parts, is the hospital liable for her traffic accidents while she is driving her own vehicle?
6. What are the steps in advancing within the ACHE organization?
7. Visit the ACHE Web site at http://www.ache.org and download the CEO employment contract that is available. Why is this an important document?
8. What are the typical rights and duties of an *ex officio* member of the board?

Part III

Doorways to the Hospital

Chapter 6

Outpatient Areas

Key Terms

Ambulatory surgery
JCAHO ambulatory standards
Medical group practice
Medical office building (MOB)
Outpatient services
PCs and PAs

Referred outpatients
Registration
Specialty clinics
Surgicenter
Urgicenter

INTRODUCTION

In the last 25 years, one of the biggest changes in the delivery of care in hospitals is the use of outpatient services. Some reasons attributed to the move toward outpatient care include the demand for shorter hospital stays by Medicare's prospective payment system, technological advancements that make delivery of complicated patient care safer and less invasive on an outpatient basis, the need for a low-cost alternative to inpatient care, and patient preference. As a result, we now see a multitude of medical, surgical, diagnostic, and rehabilitative services provided by hospitals on an outpatient basis.

In the outpatient setting, patients are registered rather than admitted. The registration process must capture accurate patient identification and billing data since there is no second chance to correct this information in the outpatient setting. In addition to collecting patient data, registration systems should determine patient eligibility for services and their insurance coverage, generate a daily outpatient schedule, and provide outpatient reports and forms. Whether a centralized or decentralized system is more efficient in handling outpatient registration depends on local hospital circumstances.

AMBULATORY SURGERY

Ambulatory surgery is defined as surgery (generally of a minor nature) that does not require the patient to remain overnight in the hospital. Ambulatory surgery may be performed in a traditional controlled hospital setting whereby patients enter and leave a unit or part of a hospital and the hospital's existing inpatient operating rooms are used. Surgery may also be performed in a separate area of the hospital campus that is designated for ambulatory surgery. This is usually called a surgicenter. Satellite surgicenters are those not located on the hospital's campus. Those that are independently operated by physicians in competition with the hospital are commonly called freestanding surgery centers.

CLINICS

Over most of the past 100 years, there has been very little change in the nature of the urban hospital clinic. There are, however, wide variations in types of clinics, ranging from an array of very sophisticated, middle-class, private physician offices to large, urban teaching hospitals manned by house staffs. In urban areas, clinics continue to serve mostly the indigent and to provide medical resources for those who do not have access to private physicians.

Hospital clinics generally follow the lines of specialization within the hospital medical staff. This means that hospitals offer outpatient clinics in medicine, surgery, obstetrics, gynecology, and pediatrics, in addition to the basic services. In the more technologically advanced and tertiary teaching centers, there can be as many as 50 or 60 different specialty clinics that are open on various days during each month. Due to the deficit financial nature of hospital clinics and emergency departments, hospital controllers and administrators try to cost-shift to third-party payers to pay a portion of the bill for indigent outpatients. Another option is the dissolution of hospital clinics through the establishment of private group practices or the sharing of services. Smart administrators of hospitals usually provide clinic space to physicians, knowing the hospital will reap profits from admissions, surgeries, diagnostic procedures, and even prescriptions.

In an attempt to make the utilization of emergency departments more appropriate, another category of delivery, known as urgent care centers, has evolved. Also called urgicenters, they provide services to nonemergency patients whose treatment needs rank between those treated in an emergency department and those receiving clinic services. Some hospitals have found it valuable to keep the urgicenter on the hospital campus as part of their emergency service. This can take the pressure of bottlenecks from the hospital's emergency department and provide the patient with much cheaper services. Many times an urgent care center may be staffed with a physician's assistant or a nurse practitioner.

ANCILLARY OUTPATIENT SERVICES

Due primarily to the great increase in emergency department visits and associated ambulatory visits, hospital supporting services—laboratory, imaging, and physical therapy—have grown considerably and now provide a major source of support for the hospital's outpatients. When patients are referred for laboratory or imaging studies or for physical therapy, rather than registering them as clinic patients, the hospital records these patients as referred outpatients. The number of patients referred to ancillary services has been on the rise, creating a significant factor in the hospital's revenue.

Freestanding imaging centers also provide the traditional services offered by hospital-based outpatient radiology services. Some of these new centers are previously existing private radiology practices with new names. In many instances, they are physician owned and may directly compete with the hospital for revenue.

GROUP PRACTICE

Medical group practice can be described as the furnishing of medical services by two or more physicians organized to provide medical care or treatment through the shared use of equipment and work staff, with the income from the medical practice distributed in a previously agreed-upon understanding. The concept of group practice in medicine began to evolve around 1900. (Though W.W. Mayo is credited with establishing the Mayo Clinic in 1864, multi-physician clinics did not really begin in earnest until the turn of the century). Prior to that time, physicians joined to practice medicine, but they did not consider themselves an organized group practice.

Groups are usually organized as single-owner groups, partnerships, professional corporations (PCs), professional associations (PAs), or foundations, usually depending on the applicable state laws. There are secondary definitions of large physician-directed multispecialty groups. As a rule, the largest growing specialty groups are the emergency department groups that contract to provide services for a hospital's emergency department and primary care service groups that are based either in the hospital itself or in the hospital's medical office building complex.

Some of the reasons physicians join a group practice are the ease of consultation; the reduction of administrative overhead and sharing call; the opportunities for physicians to recruit others into their group; financial security and incentives for the physicians; less use of hospital facilities by the physicians; improved clinical results, especially in prenatal mortality; and the tendency to improve professional competency.

MEDICAL OFFICE BUILDINGS (MOBs)

With the changing patterns of ambulatory medicine, physicians as well as hospital management have had to rethink the conventional ways of rendering service and providing resources. In many communities, the traditional office with one physician and one nurse has been rapidly disappearing. Physicians have learned that banding together in medical office buildings, sharing overhead, and, in some instances, staff and other resources such as laboratories and imaging facilities, have provided efficient and economical ways to practice outpatient medicine.

Hospitals have recognized that efficient outpatient care can be made available in a structured, well-planned medical office building. The medical office building is usually a separate building, but it could include segments of existing hospitals, such as floors, wings, or towers that have been made into medical office building suites. Medical office building concepts provide an interesting example of a winning situation where their establishment is good for the hospital, the physician, and the patient. They allow for increased efficiency in patient care on an ambulatory basis. When the building is on the hospital campus, the patient frequently receives a one-step service of quality care supported by the hospital medical staff. Viable medical office buildings permit physician groups to establish an excellent nucleus for the development of health maintenance organizations. A medical office building stabilizes the office location of key staff physicians who might shift their offices or their allegiance to other hospitals or other communities. It can also give the hospital an additional tool for physician recruiting. The presence of a viable medical office building on the hospital campus or within the hospital has been shown to increase the patient census at the hospital.

The actual organization, financial structure, and legal structure for medical office building complexes vary. There are essentially four models: 1) the hospital owns and maintains the facility; 2) the medical office building is owned by the physicians and the hospital acts as a partner to secure loans and other financial arrangements; 3) the physicians and an outside developer own the building and lease the land from the hospital; or 4) the physicians and an outside developer own the building and the hospital leases space from the physician-developer group.

STANDARDS OF ACCREDITATION

The Joint Commission on Accreditation of Healthcare Organizations (JCAHO) (discussed in Chapter 24) constantly changes, updates, and revises its standards, which now include new standards for ambulatory care areas of hospitals and free standing clinics. It is thus possible for a "doc-in-the-box" (free-standing clinic) to gain accreditation by the Joint Commission.

MAJOR GROWTH AREAS IN THE FUTURE

The future will include an even greater shift from the inpatient hospital stay to the day or ambulatory hospital concept. With this shift will be continued growth in the types and pervasiveness of alternative or substitute programs and services traditionally represented in the inpatient setting. Some examples of existing substitute programs include day chemotherapy programs, rehabilitative care programs, hospice care programs, pain intervention programs, and behavioral medicine programs. Although these programs will continue to be offered in the hospital environment, they also will be provided in separate ambulatory clinics or medical malls.

CHAPTER REVIEW

1. Why has outpatient care increased in the last 25 years?
2. What are urgicenters?
3. What is an MOB and what is its importance to a hospital?
4. What is an ambulatory surgery center (surgicenter)? Who can start and own one?
5. What is preregistration and why is it important to a hospital?
6. What is bedside registration and how is it important in customer service?
7. What is "24 hour observation" and why is it important to a hospital seeing Medicare patients?

Chapter 7

The Emergency Department

INTRODUCTION

In the early days of hospitals, the emergency room (ER) was called an accident room or accident ward. The accident room was the place to treat patients who had surgical problems because of automobile accidents, home accidents, or job-related accidents. At that time, hospital management viewed the accident room as a necessary community service but not as a glamorous hospital product. General practitioners (GPs), many specialty surgeons, obstetricians, and pediatricians had very little use for the concept of accident rooms since most of their patients were seen in the GPs' offices. Hospital interns, who were not necessarily experienced in accident situations, generally staffed accident rooms. Typically, there were registered nurses to support the interns. Things changed after World War II. As medical schools and teaching hospitals began to produce superspecialties and the general practitioner began to shrink from the medical scene, it was not long before patients discovered that they had nowhere to turn for the usual minor complaints and illnesses. The path of least resistance, and the one frequently open, was the hospital accident room or emergency room. The accident room soon became a walk-in medical clinic in most communities.

EMERGENCY DEPARTMENT UTILIZATION

For a mobile population like that of the United States, the use of the emergency department (ED) for family care has become a way of life. The relocation of families from one area to another has had a profound impact on the use of emergency departments. When an illness strikes prior to the family having had time to select a private physician, the hospital becomes the natural place to seek care.

The move of middle-income families and their physicians to suburban areas has left urban hospitals surrounded by economically disadvantaged families who depend on the hospital for medical care. However, patients who are financially able to pay for care sometimes choose emergency department services if they live a great distance from a physician's office. Many patients have learned that their medical needs may be satisfied more quickly (not always true) in hospital emergency departments. Some patients believe that emergency departments have better treatment facilities than physicians' offices. Emergency departments are used as after-hours physicians' offices and 24-hour outpatient clinics. This places a heavy burden on the facilities, space, staff, and finances of the hospital.

CATEGORIZATION OF EMERGENCY FACILITIES

Not all hospitals operate emergency departments, nor are hospitals required to do so by law, regulation, or the Joint Commission on Accreditation of Healthcare Organizations. However, if a hospital does operate an emergency service, it is held to all appropriate rules and regulations of third-party agencies. In the early 1970s, various organizations, regions, and states began to review the concept of categorizing different emergency facilities into the levels of care that they are capable of providing. State law usually designates these levels. Usually a Level 1 center is staffed with the highest level of care 24 hours per day, with nearly every specialist present in the hospital. Level ratings move down as the corresponding numbers go up, with some states designating the lowest level as Level 4 or 5. Table 7-1 describes the common standards for each level of service.

Trauma is a leading cause of death of young people in the United States. Studies have shown, however, that Level 1 trauma units may prevent many of these deaths. As a result of the studies, a few hospitals have established trauma centers, usually in large metropolitan areas. A trauma center provides high-tech emergency care to trauma victims and usually integrates with an air transport system. Most trauma centers have had an adverse financial impact on hospitals due to unpaid bills and extraordinarily high operating costs. This result has been the closing of trauma centers, particularly in urban hospitals.

Table 7-1 Levels of Emergency Service

Level 1   In large states or densely populated areas, a Level 1 emergency department usually has a specialist of every major discipline in the building 24 hours daily, and it certainly has trauma specialists. Many less populated states have lesser capabilities, but designate the few premier centers a Level 1 center. These centers may be linked with surrounding areas by helicopter or other means of rapid transportation. These are sometimes also known as trauma centers.

Level 2   A Level 2 emergency department also operates 24 hours a day, with physicians experienced in emergency care on duty in the emergency area. Specialty consultations are also available within 30 minutes.

Level 3   A Level 3 emergency department has a physician on duty 24 hours daily. Other physicians on the medical staff may be required to come in within 30 minutes when called, usually based on a rotating roster.

Level 4   A Level 4 emergency department renders life-saving first aid and makes appropriate referrals to the nearest organizations that are capable of providing more advanced services.

As previously noted in the text, these levels may vary from state to state, depending on the statutory definition—these are general guidelines.

PHYSICAL FACILITIES

It is advisable that the emergency department be located on the ground floor with easy access for patients and ambulances. In general, it is best to have the ED separate from the main entrance of the hospital. The emergency department entrance should be easily visible from the street with proper lighting and signs. It is very important that the ambulance entrance to the emergency department be large enough to admit one or more ambulances and crews negotiating the area with stretchers. Emergency departments should have waiting rooms sufficient for patients and their families and friends as well as telephone areas and restrooms close by. Imaging and laboratory services should be easily accessible to the emergency department. Oftentimes, emergency patients require imaging, and they usually need laboratory studies. If emergency departments manage a patient volume in excess of 1,000 patients per month or handle an unusually high number of fracture cases, there may be imaging facilities in the ED. A portable imaging apparatus is seldom satisfactory. If an imaging (x-ray) unit is located within the emergency department, provision must be made for the consultation services of radiology technicians and radiologists.

Generally, the emergency department has at least two or three functional areas. Typically, there is the trauma area where the severely injured surgical cases are handled. There should be a medical examining area nearby and a casting area for orthopedics. There should be observation beds for patients who need to remain in the emergency department area (for neurological and other medical reasons). These observation beds can be used during the interim before the patient moves to the inpatient nursing unit. The Committee on Trauma of the American College of Surgeons has published a model of a hospital emergency department that outlines in clear, understandable detail the proper physical facilities requirements and suggests layouts for the emergency department.

ORGANIZATION

In the organization of a hospital, the emergency department is generally considered a patient care unit under the direction of a physician, as are all patient units. However, unlike other hospital patient care units, the medical staff plays a major on-site role in the emergency department and thereby complicates the organization of the emergency department. Typically, nursing personnel staff the emergency department with nursing and auxiliary personnel as they do any other nursing unit. However, since physician coverage is usually required around the clock in the unit, there may be more of a management partnership between physicians and nurses than in other units.

The emergency department director generally reports directly to the medical staff director, to the management of the hospital, or to a committee called the emergency department committee of the medical staff. The emergency department committee is frequently made up of the medical staff that has to evaluate and plan the operations of the emergency department by enlisting the opinions and skills of a variety of people in the hospital. Typically, the emergency department committee is made up of representatives from the medical staff, nursing staff, and administration. This committee formulates the medical-administrative policies to guide the emergency department operations. It also examines the level and quality of emergency care rendered in the department. This committee may be involved in analyzing the flow of patients and the relationship of the emergency department patients to the ancillary services, such as imaging and laboratory.

ADMISSIONS

It is important to realize that the emergency department has a significant impact on the hospital's inpatient population. About one third of the hospital's admissions come through the emergency department. It is important to track these patients by physician and by payer mix.

Emergency department patients commonly follow one of five paths. The patient may 1) be treated and sent home; 2) be treated, held over in the emergency department for observation in a holding room, and then sent home; 3) require emergency surgery, go directly to the operating room, and then to an inpatient unit; 4) be admitted directly to the inpatient unit; or 5) be stabilized in the emergency department and transferred to another hospital for admission.

PHYSICIAN COVERAGE OF THE EMERGENCY DEPARTMENT

Various methods are employed to provide physician coverage for hospital emergency service. General state and federal legislation, e.g., the Emergency Medical Treatment and Active Labor Act (EMTALA), shifts in population growth, and additional emphasis on ambulatory medicine are some of the factors to be considered when selecting the proper staffing method.

Staffing Models

There are six common methods for staffing emergency departments. They are:

1. The hospital can require physicians on the medical staff to provide rotating coverage, or the hospital may permit the attending staff to provide voluntary coverage in staffing the emergency department. This allows physicians to acquire new patients who will be seen later in the physician's office.
2. The medical staff may voluntarily divide the on-call task and rotate the duty each month; the medical staff may also be used for specialty referrals from the emergency department.
3. Residents and medical students can staff the emergency department. This is common in large teaching hospitals.
4. A large group of private practitioners may contractually agree to staff the emergency department while retaining their individual practices.
5. A small group of specialty physicians may staff the emergency service under contract, and they do not maintain a private practice.
6. A hospital may employ full-time salaried physicians.

It is imperative to note that contracts for emergency department coverage give rise to legal questions and issues involving the hospital's liability for malpractice or negligence by any of the doctors. It is important that if the hospital is contracting for services, it be made clear to patients that the physicians are *independent contractors* and not employees of the hospital. This can be done with visibly posted signs and physician name tags prominently bearing the name of the physician's practice.

Since 1979, when emergency medicine became recognized as a medical specialty, hospitals have been replacing their part-time staffs with emergency specialists. Residency-trained emergency graduates of accredited programs are eligible for board certification. In order to become a board certified emergency physician, practitioners must successfully complete an examination given by the American Board of Emergency Medicine.

RECORDS

Good medical and administrative practice demands that the hospital initiate medical records on each patient visiting the emergency department. It is also necessary for the hospital to protect itself legally. Most emergency department medical records are simple compared to the extensive inpatient records. Generally, they carry administrative and basic statistical data about the patient with a place for appropriate baseline clinical data, such as blood pressure and temperature, plus a space for physicians' and nurses' notes. Generally, the emergency record is limited to a few sheets. If a patient is admitted to the hospital, the emergency service record accompanies the patient, and the record is made a part of the patient's medical chart. If the patient is not admitted, the emergency record may be retained in the emergency department, and another copy may be sent to the medical records department for proper storage. It is common practice in many emergency departments to have several copies of the medical record. Emergency personnel forward one copy to the attending physician to aid in the patient's future care, to provide continuity of care, and as a professional courtesy.

It is typical for emergency departments to maintain a register or log of patients. This is usually an appointment book or a form containing such information as the patient's name, date of admission to the emergency department, age, sex, type of medical or surgical problem, and the disposition of the case. The emergency department log provides information for analysis and studies, such as frequency of visits, the nature of the visits, etc. When patients arrive at the emergency department with a previous inpatient admission history at that hospital, the physicians and nurses treating the patient will usually request the patient's prior inpatient medical record so that proper treatment can be given. It is also important that all ED personnel know and understand the latest HIPAA (Health Insurance Portability and Accountability Act, discussed in Chapter 19) regulations.

FINANCIAL IMPLICATIONS

Because the emergency department is generally open 24 hours a day with heavy costs in the area of physician salaries and around-the-clock nursing staff, the hospital must look at the broader implications of providing emergency service. A traditional view of the emergency department is as that of a drain on hospital resources. Depending on the financial status of the outpatients visiting the department, especially in urban areas, it could be a financial drain. In an average hospital, significant portions of inpatients come through the emergency department. Studies have shown that emergency department patients are high users of ancillary services of the hospital. The high use of the ancillary services by both outpatients and inpatients contributes to the increased charge structure and improves cash flow for the hospitals.

Typically, one third of the bill for a hospital emergency patient stems from the emergency department; the remaining charges are generated through the utilization of ancillary services. With the use of ancillary services and the element of free care in the outpatient aspect of the emergency services, the financial dimension of the emergency department is complex.

It is common for urban emergency departments to run a high level of bad debts and free care. The principal factor causing this financial drain is the emergency service's third-party insurance demographics. Because of the physician availability problem in our urban areas, a large number of welfare, Medicaid, and indigent patients use the emergency service as a substitute primary care physician. In many states, the government's Medicaid outpatient reimbursement formulas do not meet the hospital's costs, thereby leaving the emergency department with a large financial deficit and inadequate cash flow.

The typical patient's bill for a visit to the emergency department may include three different types of charges. First, there is a basic charge that varies among hospitals; this is the part of the bill that helps pay for the fixed and overhead charges in the department. Second, there may be a separate charge for physicians' services. If the hospital employs the emergency department physician or the house staff is used, there may not be a separate charge for professional services. Usually the group contracting with the hospital will do their own billing. Third, there may be an ancillary or special services charge for drugs, imaging, pathology, or even anesthesia.

The emergency department must be viewed for its total hospital impact rather than as a restricted departmental outpatient center. Emergency departments may increase the hospital's census and cash flow in the inpatient area. Improved physical facilities, competent professional staffing, and the image of high quality patient care in the community all seem to add up to increased volume in the hospital's emergency departments, which then tends to lower the cost per visit.

LEGAL IMPLICATIONS

The Federal Emergency Medical Treatment and Active Labor Act (EMTALA) mandates that hospitals have a duty at least to examine and stabilize patients. If the necessary level of treatment cannot be provided, the patient should be transferred to a more appropriate facility. Failure to comply with EMTALA can jeopardize the hospital's Medicare standing.

A common legal question arising in the emergency department is the issue of treating minors who come to the emergency department without their parents or guardians. Usually, state legislation protects hospitals in this situation. Lawyers generally will advise emergency department physicians that if there is a threat to life or limb it is far better to treat the minor patient, even in the absence of securing parental consent, than to send the minor out of the emergency department.

Another important issue in the area of hospital liability is the matter of the hospital's responsibility to inform (in non-technical language) the emergency department patient about the type and timing of any recommended follow-up medical care. Many hospitals, in attempting to adopt this principle, give the patient written follow-up instructions to reduce their liability and to improve communications.

The presence of intoxicated patients in the emergency department usually creates a sense of turmoil. Such patients can be loud, hostile, demanding, and difficult to deal with. Many times the police escort these patients into the area, often from the scene of a recent accident. Frequently the police authorities ask for a blood alcohol test. This is a clinical laboratory procedure to determine the level of alcohol present in the patient's blood at any given time, the results of which could prove whether the patient is legally intoxicated. Hospital staff members should be cautious and follow their state laws.

Legally, no government hospitals and, in some jurisdictions, no hospitals receiving government financial support may refuse emergency care based on or discriminate on issues such as race, color, creed, or national origin. All hospitals participating in Medicare that have emergency departments must provide medical services to anyone needing emergency care. Patients with an unstable condition may not be transferred to another hospital without authorization from medical personnel, patient consent, and an agreement by the receiving hospital.

CHAPTER REVIEW

1. What is the leading cause of death in the United States among young people?
2. What are some functional areas of a typical emergency department?
3. What percent of admissions typically come through the ED?
4. Discuss the financial implications of an ED to the hospital.
5. Discuss EMTALA.
6. Discuss several methods of providing emergency room physician staffing.

Chapter 8

The Admitting Department

INTRODUCTION

Admitting is the process whereby an individual becomes a hospital inpatient. The admitting department has changed over the last decade. It once was a relatively easy matter for the patient or the patient's family to give the admissions clerk routine information necessary to admit the patient. Those days are gone. Hosts of external factors—the legal system, third-party payers, government regulations, and review programs—have changed the role of the admissions office. Today more and more people interact with the admissions department as an individual patient's case management has become very important to hospitals and payers under prospective payment reimbursement systems.

THE DEPARTMENT'S ROLE IN PUBLIC RELATIONS

Since the admitting department functions as an early hospital control point, it assumes a significant role in hospital public relations. Essentially, this department is responsible for forming external relationships between the hospital and patients and their families, as well as internal relationships between the hospital and admitting physicians and their office staffs. Good communication and departmental efficiency are vital to foster healthy internal and external relationships.

As the hospital doorway for patients and their families, early and often lasting impressions begin at the admitting office. A positive image can be generated through patient information booklets or brochures that are distributed either before or upon admission of the patient. Frequently, these are given to the patient's family and to visitors as well. A booklet for patients outlining the dos and don'ts will make the patient's hospital stay a bit more understandable, comfortable, and a bit less stressful.

The appearance of the waiting area is particularly important. The hospital's volunteer auxiliary staff can be instrumental in maintaining the appearance of the area, routinely straightening magazines and chairs, greeting people as they come and go, and calling for assistance when needed.

Several years ago, the American Hospital Association developed a Patient's Bill of Rights that most hospitals have adopted. It explains a hospital's obligations to patients and clarifies the relationships among the physician, the patient, and the hospital organization during the patient's stay. This Patient's Bill of Rights should be included in the patient information booklet.

In addition, patients should find the admitting staff to be sympathetic, understanding, courteous, and professional, never forgetting that patients are sick and nearly all would be somewhere else if given the choice.

The admitting department also plays a major role in sustaining positive relations with the medical staff and hospital personnel. Indeed, all who enter the department will have a perception of the hospital based on their experience with the admitting staff. Any negative experience that a patient encounters in the admitting department may adversely affect the patient's opinion of the physician and other hospital personnel, thus becoming negative public relations.

FUNCTIONS OF THE ADMITTING DEPARTMENT

Besides the admitting department's role as a key public relations arm of the hospital, the department is also responsible for beginning the processing of the patient's financial information. For example, it is involved in financial interviewing, credit arrangements, and acceptance of hospital deposits for patients without insurance. The admitting department is also involved in quality and utilization processes such as preadmission registration, preadmission testing, review of hospital admission designations, and review of length of stay. It is here that Health Insurance Portability, Accountability Act (HIPAA) (discussed in Chapter 19) confidentiality information is relayed to the patient and that advanced directives and a durable power of attorney for health care forms are offered. Other functions in the admitting department can include assigning beds, preparing the daily census, and acting as liaison with physicians' offices.

TYPES OF ADMISSIONS

It has been common practice in hospitals to classify admissions based on the patient's needs. Emergency admissions are patients who have to be immediately admitted to the hospital for life-threatening causes. When there is not a vacant inpatient bed, emergency admissions can be housed in the hospital's emergency department holding area. The next category of admission is urgent. These patients usually are admitted within 24 hours of being seen by their physician because their life or well-being could be threatened. The least critical category for admissions is elective. These patients' lives are not immediately endangered. Their admission can be delayed, sometimes with the patient being sent home to be called later when a bed is available.

The hospital's medical staff should be asked to review or to modify these admission definitions periodically. In addition, the hospital's medical staff has an obligation to review the categories of admission and define them based on local community conditions, for example, by considering the age of the population and the services available in the hospital.

PREADMISSION

Admission of a patient can be facilitated if certain tasks are handled prior to the patient being admitted to the hospital. The preadmission process involves the admissions employee receiving relevant personal and financial data with the patient's hospital reservation. This data can be obtained by mail or telephone, days in advance of the patient's actual admission. The objective of gathering preadmission data is to expedite the processing of patients into the hospital, thereby reducing waiting time in the admissions office or the lobby.

Often a hospital has developed an advanced admitting program whereby the above process is facilitated through the *physician's office* by sending the patient certain forms in advance to be completed and returned to the hospital prior to admission. The forms request the patient's name, address, certain statistical information, and details regarding the patient's financial insurance coverage. They may also ask if the patient has special requests, for example, VIP rooms or any special needs required during the hospitalization. The hospital would then have someone ready to greet the patient upon arrival and escort him/her directly to the assigned bed.

Prior to the patient's arrival for admission, certain clinical preadmission testing is conducted for many elective patients. The process of preadmission clinical testing involves the patient coming to the hospital a day in advance for ancillary studies, including laboratory tests, imaging, or electrocardiograms. The majority of these test results turn out to be normal or at least what the ordering physician expected. However, if an unexpected abnormality is discovered, the test results might delay a patient's surgery or course of treatment. The patient may remain an outpatient until the problem is handled; the patient can then enter the hospital for the surgery or other treatment. If the treatment or surgery is not delayed, the patient might have to remain in the hospital longer than necessary.

Preadmission testing has four recognized benefits for the patient, the physician, and the hospital:

1. It frequently reduces the need to postpone or cancel surgery at the last minute by discovering unusual test results prior to admission.
2. It allows the hospital's busy ancillary areas (imaging and laboratory) and surgical suite to distribute the workload more evenly.
3. It provides information to the physician prior to the admission and makes the physician's preoperative patient workup much easier.
4. Because the testing is done on an outpatient basis, it frequently shortens the length of the patient's hospital stay, thereby reducing the cost to the patient and the insurance company; it also frees beds for other patients.

Preadmission testing does have drawbacks. Sometimes the patient is too ill to go to the hospital for diagnostic studies. Obviously, preadmission will not work on emergency admissions. Some patients are unwilling or unable to leave work to go to the hospital a day or two prior to admission. Some patients find it inconvenient to travel long distances to the hospital in advance of their admission.

Third-party payers have been the leaders in preadmission testing. However, there is careful scrutiny to insure there is not test duplication between what the physician has performed in his/her office and what the physician again orders for the hospital to perform upon admission.

One benefit of the preadmission testing program is the easing of scheduling problems in the surgical suite. Operating room time must be scheduled in advance for patients who are admitted for elective surgery. With preadmission tests already accomplished before the patient is admitted, the operating room staff can better schedule its workload. The admitting department must work very closely with the operating room scheduler to coordinate the admission and the operating room time. Some hospitals allow the admitting department to schedule surgical time in the operating room, but this is not a common practice.

CONSENT FORMS

Frequently, the admitting department is responsible for obtaining a patient's signature on certain consent forms upon admission. Consent forms generally fall into two categories: 1) consent forms for general procedures and general treatment, and 2) special consent forms for any surgical or medical procedure. Usually the admitting office is responsible for the general consent forms, while the physicians and other clinical members of the medical team may be involved in obtaining signatures on the special consent forms, since they require informed consent. General consent forms often cover routine procedures such as laboratory work, imaging, or simple medical treatment. Special consent forms are involved in major or minor surgery, anesthesia, radiation therapy, or certain imaging treatments, and experimental procedures.

BED ASSIGNMENTS

Beds may be assigned to patients by patient care categories, by buildings, or by floors, depending on the institution's bed allocation policy. Traditionally, bed boards, or visual display boards, have been used to control and monitor the assignment of beds. In some hospitals, visual display boards are being replaced by computerized displays and are being integrated with hospital information systems. These must comply with HIPAA regulations.

CHAPTER REVIEW

1. What is a Patient's Bill of Rights?
2. Discuss various types of hospital admissions.
3. What is preadmission testing? What are the advantages?
4. What are patient consent forms?
5. How does the hospital's admitting department obtain needed information when a patient is an emergency unconscious admission?
6. List several things that patient consent forms must contain. What are the consequences to the hospital and to the physician if procedures are conducted and consent has not been obtained?

Part IV
The Medical Team

Chapter 9

The Medical Staff

> ## Key Terms
>
> Allied health staff
> American Medical Association
>   (AMA)
> Appointment process
> Approved residency program
> Categories of membership
> Chief resident
> Clinical department
> Clinical privileges
> Closed staff
>
> Credentials committee
> Executive committee
> Hospitalist
> Medical staff bylaws
> National Practitioner Data Bank
> National Resident Matching
>   Program
> Reappointment
> Specialty boards

INTRODUCTION

The hospital medical staff is an organized body of physicians, dentists, podiatrists, sometimes nurse midwives, nurse practitioners, physician assistants, psychologists, and in some instances, allied health staff professionals who attend patients and participate in related clinical care duties.

The medical staff has the greatest impact on the quality and quantity of care given in the hospital. The medical staff is the heart of the hospital. Members of the medical staff have been authorized by the board of trustees to treat patients in the hospital and are accountable to the governing authority. They are accountable to the hospital for high-quality patient care through the application of ethical, clinical, and scientific procedures and practices. Though the governing body has the ultimate legal and moral responsibility for the hospital, including the quality of medical care, the board of trustees cannot practice medicine and is dependent upon the members of the medical staff to admit patients, provide quality patient care, and partially police themselves.

The board of trustees appoints the medical staff. The staff formulates its own medical policies, rules, and regulations and is responsible to the board for the quality of patient care. The medical profession is a disciplined, professional group made up of highly individualistic members who have their own unique approaches to medicine and organizational relationships. Therefore, the task of coordinating the efforts of the medical staff with the board of trustees, the administrator, and the rest of the hospital can be a challenging one.

BECOMING A PHYSICIAN

The training period to become a doctor is a long and arduous one. Usually, entering medical school requires at least an undergraduate degree, with a concentration of courses in biology, chemistry, and other sciences, followed by the Medical College Admission Test (MCAT). To gain admission to an accredited, 4-year college of medicine, applicants must score competitively on the MCAT.

After graduating from medical school, it is mandatory for a newly graduated physician to complete a residency or postgraduate specialty training program in a hospital. The graduate does this by applying for the National Resident Matching Program, a program developed in 1951 by representatives from the American Association of Medical Colleges (AAMC), the American Medical Association (AMA), and various hospital associations. This group acts as a national clearinghouse for matching the preferences of new graduates with the hospitals offering residencies.

The clearinghouse function gives a greater degree of freedom of choice for both the hospital and the medical student. Before the matching plan, graduating medical school students had to negotiate their own internships or residencies with individual hospitals. Since the students were notified by a specific date, it was often too late in the year to seek alternate internships if they were turned down. The matching plan allows more students in approved residency programs (approved by the Council of Education of the AMA). Internships used to be the first year's postgraduate training for physicians. However, the internship category no longer is a part of the AMA approved programs, and the first year is now residency. The results of the matching plan are announced early each spring.

A hospital that has an approved residency program is more complex and perhaps more interesting than a hospital that does not offer educational programs. The teaching hospital is essentially a living classroom. In these teaching hospitals, the residents are referred to by their years of training. For example, a first-year resident is called a postgraduate year 1 resident, or PGY1. Therefore, a PGY1 would be a low person on the resident (house staff) totem pole; he/she is under the guidance of a senior resident who, in turn, is under the guidance of the chief resident in a given specialty. The chief residents in each specialty have the supervisory, managerial, and teaching responsibilities in the program. Generally, these residents are not licensed physicians, though in many states special temporary licenses are granted to practice within the institution that has the approved residency program. There was a time when the residents worked for a meager stipend. Now the residents receive respectable salaries for their efforts. The residents learn a great deal at the hospital, but they also give the hospital considerable patient services in return.

After physicians complete their hospital residency programs, many seek to become certified in their specialties. This may require further training. Certification, referred to as board certification, is under the jurisdiction of special boards such as the American Board of Surgery. The objective of specialty boards and associations is to upgrade the qualifications of specialists. These boards and associations have increased the length of time needed for training, developed subspecialties, and sponsored numerous continuing education programs and professional journals. After rigorous examinations and proven abilities and practice, certification by a specialty board is indeed recognition of professional competency. Fellowship in a specialty college is also meaningful peer recognition of competence.

There has been a movement toward recertification by specialty boards in an attempt to ensure that physicians maintain an acceptable level of qualifications in their specialties. For instance, certification by the American Board of Surgery is valid for 10 years. Physicians may apply for recertification as long as they are active, hold privileges in a hospital accredited by JCAHO, and have received satisfactory evaluations by the medical director. Those who pass the examination given by the American Board of Surgery are recertified.

CONTINUING MEDICAL EDUCATION

Following appointment to the medical staff of the hospital, the physician is obligated to provide proof of participation in a program of continuing medical education (CME). JCAHO and all state medical organizations stipulate that the medical staff participate in programs of continuing education. The scope and complexity of a physician's individual continuing education program will be left to the physician, but must meet the needs of the hospital's in-house medical staff credentialing program. This usually varies depending on the resources at hand and the needs of the hospital, which is directly relevant to the type of patient care delivered at the hospital. CMEs of each staff member are documented and placed in that member's medical staff file.

ORGANIZED MEDICINE

In 1847, some 250 physicians, representing more than 40 medical societies and 28 colleges from 22 states, came together and founded the AMA. Pressure to begin the AMA stemmed from the poor quality of medical education in the United States at that time, the very brisk traffic in patent medicines and secret remedies, and the questionable ethics of many physicians of the time. The people who founded the AMA believed that a national association of physicians was needed to lead the crusade for improved medical education and patient care. The founding objectives of the AMA were generally to promote the science and art of medicine to promote better health for all people.

The AMA is involved in the legislative process and has become part of a strong hospital and medical lobby. In order to respond effectively to the regulatory and legal environment, the AMA has enhanced its original mission to include formulating national health care policies.

MEDICAL STAFF ORGANIZATION

The internal organization of the medical staff varies from hospital to hospital. Complex university or teaching hospitals differ from the smaller community hospitals. Because of the efforts of the JCAHO and its accreditation standards, the differences are less extensive today than in the past. The standards stipulate that there is to be a single organized medical staff that has overall responsibility for the quality of the professional services provided by individuals with clinical privileges, as well as accountability to the governing body.

Appointment to the medical staff is a formal process that is outlined in each hospital's medical staff bylaws, with encouragement for standardization from the JCAHO. A brief outline of a typical appointment process that a doctor must go through is:

1. The applying physician completes a written application that includes information about his or her education, privileges at other hospitals, recommendations, years of practice, lawsuits, etc. The completed application is usually forwarded to the hospital CEO.
2. The application is reviewed for completeness, all items are verified, and a check is made with the National Practitioner Data Bank (discussed later in this chapter). The application is then sent for screening to the head of the specific department or specialty (e.g., medicine or surgery) to which the physician is applying.
3. The application is then forwarded to the medical staff's credentials committee, which reviews the physician's qualifications and past professional

performance. It is at this point that the credentials committee may request a meeting with the applicant.

4. The executive committee for the medical staff reviews and discusses the application. It sends its recommendation on to the hospital's governing body.

5. The board of trustees or one of its committees reviews the application. The board will accept, reject, or defer the application. If the application is questionable, requires more information, or needs discussion, it may be referred to the joint conference committee.

6. The CEO usually notifies the physician that the appointment has been approved or rejected. The notice letter sent to the physician also notes any limitations on privileges requested. In receiving approval, a physician is granted certain clinical privileges (procedures the doctor is permitted to perform within the hospital). This is called the individual's privilege delineation. The privilege delineation process is based on verifiable information made available to the credentials committee. A physician's current competence in his or her discipline is the crucial determination of privileges. The privileges are recorded, and the record is kept on file in key places within the hospital—for example, within the emergency department, in the operating room, and in the medical staff office.

The physician who has applied to the medical staff and been admitted is appointed in two separate categories of membership: 1) to a clinical department such as surgery, obstetrics, pediatrics, or urology, and 2) with a status based on the *extent* of the physician's *participation* in the hospital. Staff membership status may be categorized as explained in Figure 9-1.

The organization of the hospital medical staff is divided into medical specialty departments and sections. For example, there may be departments of medicine, surgery, obstetrics and gynecology, and pediatrics. In larger hospitals, these departments may be further subdivided into sections. Each clinical department has a physician designated as chief or director who is the medical administrative head. This person is generally selected through a process outlined in the medical staff bylaws. Usually this is done through election of departmental members or by appointment by the hospital board of trustees.

CLOSED AND OPEN MEDICAL STAFFS

Historically, individual hospitals have controlled their own admissions to their medical staff. A closed medical staff is one in which the medical *staff* closely monitors and restricts any new applicants to the medical staff or to a department of the medical staff. This is generally done with the concurrence of the hospital

Active or attending staff—These medical staff members have full rights and privileges. Each physician with this designation may be required to admit a certain number of patients each year or they lose active privileges. This will reduce the number of physicians who may wish to be on the medical staff of every hospital and not truly support the hospital.

Associate staff—Medical staff members have incomplete privileges and may be working toward active staff designation. They may have to be in this designation for a number of months while their colleagues evaluate their care, or they may have a limited number of admissions per month.

Provisional staff—These may be new staff members; there may be a probationary period associated with this . . . often they are supervised by other physicians for a certain number of cases.

Courtesy staff—A hospital may classify a physician as a courtesy staff member if that physician does not often admit patients to that hospital.

Consulting staff—These physicians do not admit patients, but rather they are called in to consult on particular patients who have been admitted by other physicians.

Temporary staff—These physicians are given privileges for a designated time, usually to treat one patient.

Figure 9-1 Status of medical staff membership.
The above are general guidelines. The governing document for the hospital that will determine the level of medical staff membership is the medical staff bylaws—this document will be different for each hospital, determined by which medical staff members write the bylaws and what changes the board of directors or trustees makes to the document. Physicians should seek legal guidance, as many antitrust issues can arise.

board of trustees. When a hospital does permit a closed medical staff, it is usually based upon considerations related to the quality of and need for patient care within the hospital and within the community. There may also be closed medical staffs within selected departments or sections in the hospital—three notable examples are the imaging, emergency, and pathology departments. In these hospital-based departments, the hospital signs a contractual agreement with a physician or a professional group to allow exclusive services in the department. The courts have generally found this to be a legal arrangement if such agreements are based upon significant medical and administrative considerations. Closed medical staff issues are frequently addressed in the courts under the federal antitrust laws. Additionally, since the Federal Trade Commission (FTC) has the power to promulgate rules and regulations defining unfair practices in this area, it is reasonable to assume that it will be a predominant enforcement agency relative to medical staff admissions in years to come. An open staff essentially admits all qualified physicians who meet the hospital's guidelines.

MEDICAL STAFF COMMITTEES

The JCAHO standards dictate that the medical staff will develop bylaws to self-govern and to be accountable to the governing body. The medical staff conducts its business through committees. The committee chairpersons are either selected by members of the staff or appointed by the president of the staff.

One of the most important committees is the medical staff executive committee. Generally, the executive committee is composed of officers of the medical staff and a number of elected members from the staff. Typically, this committee meets monthly, conducting the business of the medical staff. The hospital CEO usually attends. The medical executive committee coordinates various committees and promulgates rules that affect the different clinical departments of the staff. The credentials committee, the medical records committee, the tissue committee, and the medical audit and quality committee are other key committees of the staff. The credentials committee has the responsibility to review the qualifications of new physicians applying for membership. This committee also reviews the credentials of medical staff members who must be reappointed. Reappointment is usually either once a year or every other year. It is a review to insure that the reapplying physician has attended committee meeting, has not been involved in lawsuits, is getting on well with his or her peers and the hospital employees, and has renewed his or her medical insurance coverage and renewed training certificates such as CPR. The credentials committee could also be the committee to investigate breaches of ethics or misconduct among the members of the medical staff. This committee reports directly to the executive committee.

Usually, a medical quality improvement committee is the principal instrument for review of quality improvement matters, e.g., patient and surgical outcomes, the number of cesarean sections, etc. It also reviews the quantity and quality of patient records as written by physicians, nurses, or other associated health professionals in the hospital. It also serves as a monitor of the physicians who have delinquent medical records. This committee generally works closely with the hospital's medical records administrator.

An efficient medical audit committee and a well-functioning tissue committee traditionally have been key instruments in assessing quality. The tissue committee provides a vehicle to confirm the diagnosis for surgical cases and acts as a control for unnecessary surgery. Practicing surgeons plus a member of the hospital pathology department make up the membership. The tissue committee reviews all surgical cases to determine, based on the review of tissue taken from the patient, whether the surgery was necessary. Tissue removed from an operation is forwarded to the pathology laboratory for postoperative diagnosis and review.

THE MEDICAL DIRECTOR

The medical staff sometimes elects a part-time medical director, or sometimes the hospital employs one full-time or part-time. Generally, the medical director is a top-level management employee. If the medical director works part-time in that position, he or she may also see patients, and therefore could be a member of the medical staff. The medical director's role is to evaluate clinical performance and to enforce hospital policy related to quality care. However, as in other management jobs, the role may be expanded to include other activities. This person can be an excellent liaison between the administrator and the medical staff, being able to speak doctor to doctor.

THE HOSPITALIST

A phenomenon of the last 10 years has been the addition of a hospitalist to the medical staff. This physician (or these physicians) is usually an internal medicine specialist who makes daily rounds and visits every patient in the hospital. The advantages are many—among them, the physician, by limiting his/her practice to the hospital, clearly understands the inner workings of the hospital better than physicians who also have an office practice and must use precious time driving back and forth daily to see their patients. The hospitalist takes over the care of other physicians' patients, allowing those physicians to maximize their office time. The hospitalist contacts the physicians to report to them the condition of their hospitalized patients. This person can help to minimize the time a patient spends in the hospital by seeing each patient more frequently and by better understanding the services each department in the hospital delivers, as well as the personality of each specialized employee—those in respiratory, lab, imaging, etc. The hospitalist adds efficiency.

ALLIED HEALTH PERSONNEL

There continues to be an increasing number of nonphysicians applying for clinical privileges within the hospital, including but not limited to podiatrists, chiropractors, physician assistants, nurse practitioners, nurse midwives, and psychologists. By applying for medical staff privileges, some of these groups have raised the question of how they fit into the hospital medical staff.

Historically, with the backing of laws and regulations, hospitals have usually excluded these groups from practicing within the hospital. Generally, state regulations regarding nurse practitioners and physician assistants indicate that a physician must supervise their work. The American Medical Association agrees with the American Hospital Association on this issue and feels that full medical staff privileges should be restricted to physicians and dentists. The JCAHO has been somewhat more liberal with regard to podiatrists and has delineated what it believes a podiatrist can do within a hospital. The JCAHO permits other duly licensed health care professionals to practice in hospitals under the supervision of a practitioner who has clinical privileges. The case law on the privilege question is not clear, and it is reasonable to assume that each individual issue may be decided based upon state statutes and license practice laws within each state.

LEGAL RESTRICTIONS ON PHYSICIANS

Today, physicians are legally and professionally restricted in their practice of medicine and in their commercial ventures. Physicians' professional conduct is monitored closely, too. The Health Care Quality Improvement Act of 1986 set up a National Practitioner Data Bank in 1990 to prevent physicians, as well as other health care professionals, from hiding acts of malpractice and professional misbehavior by moving to other states. Sources of data include hospitals, malpractice insurers, and state licensing boards. Hospitals must check the data bank during their credentialing process.

A Final Word Regarding Physicians

The administrator should never forget that nothing happens in a hospital unless physicians admit patients. Without patients, the beds sit empty and the hospital employees are idle—physicians are one of the hospital's most important resources.

CHAPTER REVIEW

1. What are some items that the credentials committee typically reviews?
2. Who appoints members of the medical staff?
3. Discuss the appointment procedure to become a medical staff member of a typical hospital.
4. What are the two typical categories of medical staff membership and the six levels of admitting privileges?

5. What is the difference between a closed medical staff and an open medical staff?
6. List and discuss five medical staff committees.
7. What are the typical functions of the medical director?
8. What is a hospitalist and what role does he or she play?
9. What is the National Practitioner Data Bank?
10. Discuss the process of becoming a physician beginning with college.
11. Discuss five types of allied health personnel and their roles in the health community.

Chapter 10

Nursing Services

INTRODUCTION

Inpatients or outpatients should receive quality, courteous, and considerate care from skilled, understanding personnel. The primary department required to meet this goal is the nursing service department. Nurses account for the single largest health professional group in the country.

EARLY TRADITIONS

The early history of nursing was influenced by both individuals (e.g., Florence Nightingale) and institutions such as the Roman Catholic Church and the military. Perhaps the best-known person associated with the history of nursing is Nightingale, whose work during the Crimean War gave nursing a more respectable image. She became known as the mother of modern nursing. After the war,

Nightingale founded the Florence Nightingale Nursing School in connection with St. Thomas Hospital in London in 1859.

Records of schools for training American nurses can be traced as far back as 1798. However, American schools that embodied the principles of Florence Nightingale's school in London were established much later. The first such school was the New England Hospital for Women and Children founded in Boston in 1872. This was followed in 1873 by the Bellevue Hospital School of Nursing in New York City and the Massachusetts General Hospital in Boston school of nursing. Over the next 50 years, there were some 2,000 nursing schools established in the United States. These schools' programs include a few remaining diploma programs based in hospitals, 2-year associate degree programs in community colleges, and 4-year baccalaureate programs in colleges and universities.

NURSING EDUCATION

Changes in the well-established Nightingale nursing education model emerged following World War II. With the acute shortage of professional registered nurses (RNs), the licensed practical or vocational nurse (LPN or LVN) came into vogue. The number of nurses' aides also continued to rise. Meanwhile, educational programs for the registered nurses changed, especially in the 1960s. During this time, the 2- to 3-year hospital-diploma nursing education programs began to be phased out due to pressure on hospitals to trim budgets and pressure from the American Nurses Association for a baccalaureate or associate degree education.

Nurses now have a variety of education/experience combinations from which to select (see Table 10-1). Registered nurses can earn a PhD, which usually takes more than 7 years of academic work interspersed with practical experience. Nurses with advanced degrees may work as clinical nurse specialists, nurse clinicians, nurse practitioners, nurse midwives, or nurse anesthetists. On the other hand, a prospective nurse may choose a 1-year academic program integrated with practical experience. These nurses are called licensed practical or vocational nurses (LPNs or LVNs).

All professional and practical nurses must be licensed by the state in which they practice nursing. Every state determines its own eligibility criteria for licensing and relicensing and is responsible for suspending and revoking licenses. Usually completed educational requirements and the passing of the state's board examination are necessary for initial licensing. Relicensing can be simply achieved by payment of a small fee, if it is done before the original license expires.

There are two large and influential national professional nursing association groups. The American Nurses Association (ANA), founded in 1896, is a federa-

Table 10-1 Educational Requirements for Nurses

Educational level	Training required beyond high school	Curriculum	Training site
Registered nurse— PhD and DNS (Doctor of Nursing Science)	3 to 5 years postbac- calaureate	Academic program integrated with practical work throughout the years	University
Registered nurse— master's degree	5 to 6 academic years	1- to 2-year academic program integrated with practical work	University, hospital, and community health agencies
Registered nurse— baccalaureate degree	4 years and summer sessions	4-year academic program integrated with practical experience	University, hospital, health agencies
Registered nurse— diploma	27-36 months	1 year of academic work, 2 years of practical experience with clinical courses	Hospital
Registered nurse— associate degree	2 years	2-year academic program integrated with practical experience	Junior college
Licensed practical or vocational nurse (LPN or LVN)	1 year	1-year academic program integrated with practical experience	Vocational technical school and hospital

tion of 54 constituent associations, including those in the 50 states, the District of Columbia, and Puerto Rico. As a group, they promote legislation and speak out for nurses on legislative action programs. The other influential nursing associa- tion is the National League for Nursing (NLN) founded in 1951. This is a com- munity-centered group that brings people in the health and welfare fields together with the lay community to work primarily for the improvement of nursing service and nursing education. The NLN's membership is composed of registered nurses, practical nurses, nurses' aides, doctors, and hospital administrators—all of whom have a professional interest in nursing.

DEPARTMENT ORGANIZATION

Approximately 40 to 50 percent of all hospital employees work in the nursing department. The nursing department is organized in a pyramid fashion very much like the entire hospital. The primary responsibility rests with the director of the nursing department or division. The director is referred to as the director of nurses (DON), chief nursing officer, chief nursing executive, or now more often, as the vice president of nursing. Directors are usually selected because of their management abilities; they are often registered nurses with advanced degrees (sometimes in the specific discipline of nursing service administration). Often, the director has one or two assistant directors to aid in the management of the department. The title of supervisor is frequently given to the registered nurse who supervises or directs the activities of two or more nursing units. The supervisor may manage and direct the many nursing service activities during the evenings, nights, or weekends; thus, the titles of night supervisor, weekend supervisor, or day supervisor are often applied. The training function of the nursing department is usually assigned to a nurse carrying the title of nurse educator who is responsible for the education, orientation, and continuing in-service education of all employees in the department of nursing. This person often conducts patient education.

The nursing department is also organized along geographical lines. Each of the nursing department responsibilities for patient care is decentralized to a specific location in the hospital called a nursing unit or more commonly now, a patient care unit. Certain responsibilities and functions required to operate a nursing unit are assigned to a nurse manager. A nurse manager supervises the personnel in a patient care unit. This person may also be referred to by other titles, such as patient care manager. This person is accountable for the quality of the nursing care on the unit (medical/surgical, OB, ICU, ED, etc.), controls the supplies, and schedules the staff's working hours. Usually the nurse manager has a group of staff nurses who are assigned specific responsibilities for the nursing care of patients on the patient care unit.

A large number of employees in nursing include nurses' aides, orderlies, and technicians. These auxiliary nursing personnel commonly go through at least a hospital orientation training program before assuming their nursing duties with patients. Some states require a formal training program for nurses' aides. They do not need to be graduates of a formal education program, nor are they licensed or certified. The graduate nurse, staff nurse, or nurse manager generally assigns duties to the nurses' aides.

Many of the individual nursing units have a host of clerical functions to be performed. Unit clerks or ward clerks assigned to the nursing service handle the enormous quantity of administrative work such as coordinating reports, orders, and prescription orders for patients, answering telephones, directing visitors, helping with hospital requisitions for patients and supplies, and performing a multitude of other duties. These clerks usually work directly under the supervision of a nurse manager.

THE PATIENT CARE UNIT

As noted earlier, the nursing care of the hospital is organized in a decentralized fashion into patient care units or nursing units. The size of patient care units varies. They can be very small, with 8- to 10-bed units for specialized care, or they can be large, with 60- to 70-bed units. Perhaps the most common size is between 20 and 40 beds per unit. Nursing units generally operate in three shifts to cover a 24-hour period. They usually operate as a day shift from 7:00 a.m. to 3:00 p.m. The evening shift, called the evening tour, runs from 3:00 p.m. to 11:00 p.m., and the night shift runs from 11:00 p.m. to 7:00 a.m. Some units operate on two 12-hour shifts—7 a.m. to 7 p.m. and from 7 p.m. to 7 a.m.

Most rooms are semiprivate and accommodate two patients. There are also private or single-bed rooms. In each nursing unit, there is usually at least one single-bed room that is designed and reserved for patients with illnesses warranting isolation.

The size of the patient care unit and the distribution of single and multi-bed rooms are considered before a unit is built. Consideration is given to the cost of construction of the unit, the duplication of equipment, and how much nursing service time will be required to staff the unit. If the unit is spacious and rooms are distributed at a distance from the central nursing point, the staff must continually travel to reach a patient and supplies. Although the unit may look pleasing, it may not be work efficient. There are a variety of designs and configurations for patient care units. Some of the more common nursing unit layouts are shown in Figure 10-1. Figures 10-2 and 10-3 show the typical layouts for critical care units. Whether a rectangular or circular configuration is used, it is imperative that patients can be seen from the nursing station. Usually the patient rooms are cubicles with curtains or rooms with glass walls.

Where the patient rooms are private or semiprivate, they will vary in size. This is most often dictated by state regulation. The patient-to-nurse ratio is also affected by state regulation. For example, in January 2005, California initiated a ratio of no more than five patients to every nurse.

Other Components of the Patient Care Unit

Among the fundamentals found on patient care units is the nurses' station, which tends to be the focal point of administrative activity. The nurses' station is normally where the nurses keep their records, and it is centrally located to all the

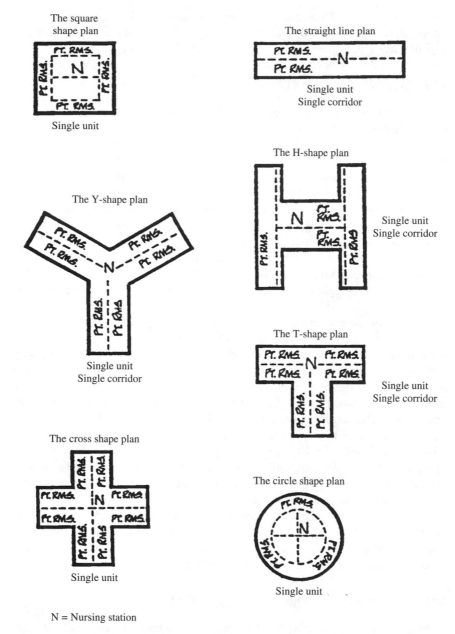

Figure 10-1 Various shapes of floor plans with alternative designs.

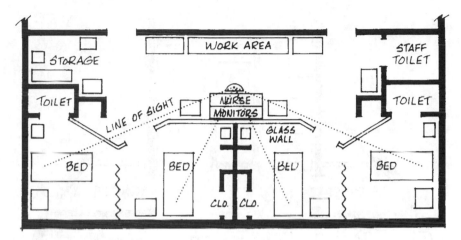

Figure 10-2 Nursing station floor plan in rectangular configuration

activities of the entire nursing unit. On a nursing unit, there is also a medicine preparation room area. Every nursing unit has a utility room. This is a workspace where clean supplies, instruments, equipment, and used or dirty items that have been utilized by the patients are stored. Usually there is a small pantry or sometimes even a large kitchen on the patient care unit, depending on the delivery method used by the hospital's dietary services department. If the food is prepackaged or preplated before coming to the patient care unit, a smaller pantry will suffice. If the food is delivered to the patient care unit in bulk fashion and distributed, a larger kitchen may be necessary. There is also a nurses' lounge where nurses take breaks, eat meals, receive in-service training, and give change-of-shift reports. Other rooms that might be found on nursing units are a common toilet/bath area, a consultation room where physicians and the families of the patients meet, and treatment rooms. Some units may also have a pleasant place for visitors to sit down with the patients outside of their rooms.

SPECIAL CARE UNITS

Special care units have developed with increased technology and modern medical advances. Over the last decade, special care units have multiplied and matured. The sophisticated modern hospital may have a variety of special care facilities to manage and maintain patients with special illnesses and injuries.

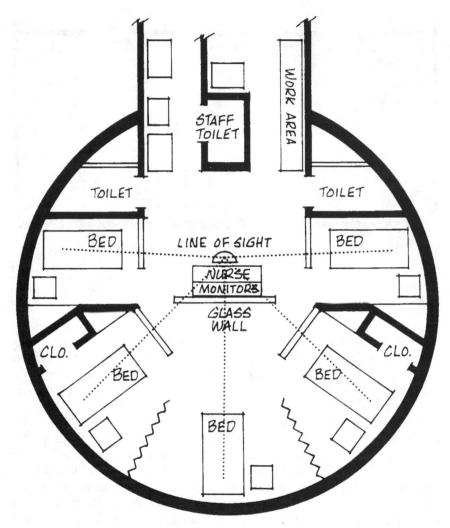

Figure 10-3 Nursing station floor plan in circular configuration.

These facilities may include intensive care units for medicine and surgery, special cardiac care units, hemodialysis or renal dialysis centers, inpatient psychiatric units, inpatient alcoholic and drug addiction units, pediatric units, and skilled nursing facilities for long-term care. A special unit need not be based in the hospital; it may be constituted as a hospital home-care program or a hospice.

Intensive Care Units

The most common type of special care unit in the hospital is the general medical/surgical intensive care unit (ICU). The ICU units were established to meet clinical demands of the hospitalized patients and their physicians. Their purpose is to manage the critically ill patient who is in a precarious clinical status and requires intense supervision. The ICUs handle both surgical and medical cases. For example, ICU cases could be patients in shock, stroke victims, or persons with heart failures, serious infections, respiratory distress, and so forth. The establishment of separate ICU units in hospitals was a major step forward in modern hospital care. By marshalling the hospital's resources in one geographic area, it is much easier to provide efficient, high quality care. Not only are sophisticated equipment and instrumentation available in ICUs, but a highly concentrated nursing staff is also used; sometimes there is one nurse to one patient. These nursing personnel may have successfully completed critical care training at the hospital and have had medical and surgical nursing care work experience.

A special offshoot of the ICU is the neonatal intensive care unit, which specializes in the management of critical health problems in the newborn. Caring for the critically ill newborn requires a specially trained nurse and physician. The neonatal intensive care units have had great success in the care of premature infants.

Coronary Care Units

The intensive care units in hospitals gave birth to coronary care units (CCUs). The CCUs may be quite familiar to the ordinary health care consumer since they have grown in popularity. Today nearly all of the medical-surgical hospitals in the United States have some CCU capacities, if one includes those facilities that have CCU capacities in their ICUs.

The CCUs do for cardiac patients what the ICUs do for severe medical and surgical patients. The CCU has had a dramatic impact on saving lives. Better CCUs and better preventive care has resulted in heart disease dropping to the number two killer in 2005, now behind cancer.

For both ICUs and CCUs, it is usual to have a cardiologist assigned full-time, part-time, or rotating to manage the units medically. Attending physicians manage their own patients. However, because of the presence of the specialist, the attending physicians no longer have total and complete control over their patients; they must realize that their care is a shared responsibility in these two units.

The nurse's role in these units is critical. The nurse should be an intelligent observer, and he or she must be able to interpret changes in a patient. Under critical circumstances, the nurse may have to diagnose and provide immediate care to the patient. One of the primary objectives of the CCU is to detect early signs of impending cardiac distress so that it may be treated before cardiac arrest takes place.

Nonacute Special Care Units

There are varieties of special care units that are not geared for life-threatening situations. One of the best examples is the renal dialysis centers that have been increasing in number over the last decade. The renal dialysis centers provide artificial kidney support for patients whose kidneys have stopped functioning properly. These units, unlike the CCUs and ICUs, provide long-term care needs for patients. Other nonacute special care units include psychiatric units and inpatient alcohol and drug-related units.

Long-Term Care Facilities

With the aging population and the number of patients who need nursing home care after hospitalization, many hospitals have become involved in long-term care programs. More and more hospitals have long-term or nursing home beds or hospital-based nursing facilities near their institutions. This can be an effective strategy to assist in discharging the patient from an acute care setting.

The patients in these facilities are generally recovering from strokes, severe orthopedic accidents, or severe medical illnesses. There are two generally recognized kinds of nursing homes or kinds of care: 1) skilled nursing facilities (SNFs) and 2) lower-level nursing facilities called intermediate care facilities (ICFs).

MODES OF NURSING CARE DELIVERY

Today there are four commonly used modes of nursing delivery: 1) case nursing, 2) functional nursing, 3) team nursing, and 4) primary care nursing.

Case Nursing

The case method of nursing is one of the earliest forms of nursing care. In this system, the nurse or case manager individually plans and administers the care of a patient. This is done on a one-to-one basis. The case method has persisted over the years in a couple of nursing areas. It is used today as the model of nursing in nursing schools because it allows nursing students to be taught an idealized patient care system. It is also used in acute care settings, such as intensive care, and may be used on the general nursing unit in private-duty nursing situations.

Functional Nursing

Starting in the 1920s and continuing into the 1940s, nurses became aware of the studies and developments in the functional division of labor in industry, as seen in the assembly line approach to manufacturing used by Henry Ford and other industrialists. Nurses then applied these time and motion studies to their own discipline. Essentially, functional nursing uses a pyramid organization to look at the division of labor. Under such an arrangement, technical aspects of each nursing staff member's job are identified, and based on this technical expertise, each unit member is given specific functions or tasks to perform on the unit. For example, one nurse might administer medications, another would give all of the treatments, a third might take all the temperatures and blood pressures of patients, and a fourth might prepare those patients going to surgery or imaging. All would give baths, make beds, and try to meet the patient's psychological and emotional needs. The simpler tasks would be given to the less trained nursing personnel and the more complex tasks to the registered nurses. Functional nursing is often utilized on the evening and night shifts where the number of tasks is generally reduced.

Team Nursing

Team nursing began around World War II when there was a growing shortage of registered nurses (RNs). In the absence of RNs, hospitals had to use technicians, vocational nurses, and nurses' aides. Frequently, the less trained nursing personnel were put under the supervision of a more highly trained registered nurse, who was called the team leader. This team was asked to provide care to a group of patients on the nursing unit. Ideally, the team leader was the best prepared person and was expected to facilitate the team in formulating and carrying out the nursing care plans for every patient assigned to the team. Team nursing fits well into the pyramid structure of the hospital organization.

Primary Care Nursing

Primary care nursing has some of the characteristics of the case method of nursing, in that one registered nurse is assigned to each patient. However, unlike the case method of nursing, the nurse assigned to the patient is not responsible only for one shift of work. The primary care nurse is responsible for the care of the patient for 24 hours a day, seven days a week. It is the primary care nurse's responsibility to assess a patient's nursing needs. The primary care nurse collaborates with other health professionals, including the physician, and formulates a plan of nursing care for which the nurse becomes responsible and accountable.

The primary care nurse provides all of the patient's custodial care needs such as bathing and feeding, as well as the patient's skilled care needs such as the administration of medications. The primary care nurse may delegate certain responsibilities for executing that plan on the other shifts, but the delegation is accomplished by means of other nursing care plans, including written notes and recordings. Carrying out the plan is never done through a supervisor or third party; thus an important element of primary care nursing is the triple A nurse. The triple A nurse is *autonomous*, is in *authority*, and is held *accountable* for the nursing care of the patient.

TERMS AND STANDARDS

An understanding of precisely which nursing standard was utilized when the nursing department's budget and staffing schedule was established is an important element in nursing service. A nursing standard or nursing norm is defined as the amount of time and resources needed or considered desirable for each patient in a 24-hour period in order to give the type of care judged appropriate. The American Hospital Association and the National League for Nursing identified various nursing standards as early as 1950. Nursing managers should ask such questions as: Is the ratio of registered nurses to other personnel in the department too high? Are there too many or too few licensed practical nurses for the situation? Is there another way to assign duties in order to improve budgetary performance? Financial managers should know that when nursing service expenses are low or below budget, a detailed look at the nursing staff patterns may be required. The following possibilities must be considered: 1) Perhaps student nurses have been utilized in place of staff nurses. 2) Perhaps nurses were attached to some other cost center and were used in place of regular staff nurses. 3) Perhaps inadequate information was available at the time the budget was established. 4) Perhaps the department was unable to fill all budgeted positions. 5) Perhaps the on-duty nursing staff is carrying an unfair load. To analyze all of these specific circumstances, a financial manager must have an understanding of certain nursing definitions and terms that are widely accepted in the nursing service area.

The patient must be able to rely on a reasonable standard of care, which is that the care the hospital renders will meet regulatory requirements and reasonable standards.

STAFFING

Nurse staffing is the result of determining the appropriate number of full-time equivalent nursing personnel (FTEs) by each nursing skill class (RNs, LPNs, nurses' aides) to operate properly each nursing unit. Given the great contrast in the levels of nursing care required by different patients, and the large labor needs of a nursing unit, staffing is a challenge for a nursing department. The key to determining how much staff and what proper qualifications are needed is found by using patient acuity systems.

Patient acuity systems classify patients into care categories and quantify the nursing effort required. Generally, a patient's physical, technical, psychological, social, and teaching requirements are assessed in determining acuity levels. A common type of classification system is a list of critical indicators or condition indicators, such as sensory deficit, oxygen therapy, and wound care, that are separately rated and then summed up to determine the patient's care category. Care categories include routine care, moderate care, complete care, and continuous care. For each patient care category, the total nursing care time is quantified by the nursing department.

Many patient acuity systems are computerized. Daily, weekly, and seasonal variations must be considered in staffing arrangement. Hospitals may use float nurses, part-time nursing pool personnel, and agency contracted nurses (rent-a-nurse) in addition to the hospital's full-time nursing staff to meet patient care needs.

SCHEDULING

Once the nursing department agrees on the standards to be used to staff the nursing unit, and the nursing administration agrees on the type of nursing (nursing modalities) best suited for the hospital, the challenge to nursing then is to schedule nursing personnel so that the patients receive the necessary care at the time they require it. Nurse scheduling is defined as determining when each member of the nursing staff will be on duty and on which shift each will work. Scheduling should take into account weekends, length of an individual's work stretches, and nursing requests for vacation and time off. Scheduling is typically done for a period of 4 or 6 weeks, and the scheduling is frequently tailored to each individual nursing unit. There are three commonly used approaches to nurse scheduling: the traditional, the cyclical, and the computer-aided traditional approaches.

Traditional Scheduling

In traditional scheduling, the nurse schedulers initiate each work period (e.g., week or month). The nurse manager makes the scheduling decisions by taking a computer keyboard or pencil and paper and looking at the roster of personnel who are available to work on specified dates and for certain durations. A great deal of responsibility is placed in the nurse manager's hands to ensure the quality and quantity of coverage on the nursing unit. The major advantage of this traditional approach is flexibility. Nurses are able to adjust to changes of environment on the patient care unit quickly. Some disadvantages of traditional scheduling include spottiness in coverage at certain times and uneven quality of coverage. Unless policies in the nursing administration leave some elasticity in the process, uneven staffing could also lead to maximum personnel cost or at the other extreme, minimum patient care.

Cyclical Scheduling

Cyclical scheduling is a system that covers a certain period of time, perhaps 1 or 3 months. This block of time is the cycle or scheduling period. Once the nurse agrees on a definite period, the scheduling in the cycle simply repeats itself period after period. The advantage of cyclical scheduling is that it provides even coverage with a higher quality of coverage determined for each nursing unit. Special requests would interfere with the coverage, which could affect the quality of staffing. The major disadvantage to cyclical scheduling is that it is inflexible compared to the traditional system and is not able to adjust rapidly to changes in the nursing unit environment. The ability to adjust is important, since change characterizes so many nursing units. The environment in which cyclical scheduling seems to work best is one in which the number of patients and their needs are fairly constant and the nurses are stable and do not rotate between shifts. New nurses can be hired into any open cyclical slot with very little difficulty.

Computer-Aided Traditional Scheduling

The third approach to scheduling uses a computer to assist in the traditional method of scheduling by applying mathematical programming. This system provides more flexibility and also reduces the operating costs involved in calculating and in working with the schedule. To some extent, a computer centralizes the scheduling process. If mathematical models are properly used, a computer can produce high-quality schedules. The system will also facilitate the incorporation of standard personnel policies into the schedule, and the policies can be applied uniformly over all nursing units. It will also add more stability to the entire nursing department. The advantages of computerized scheduling are most dramatically apparent in situations where nurses rotate frequently among shifts and where nursing environments are subject to persistent change. Computer-aided, centralized schedules minimize the time spent preparing and maintaining schedules.

TELEMONITORING AND BEDSIDE TERMINALS

Along with burgeoning technological innovation and the use of patient acuity levels, telemonitoring equipment, bedside terminals, and automated clinical records are being used by nurses. Telemonitoring equipment may vary from hospital to hospital depending on the complexity of the unit, the needs of the patients, and the resources of the hospital. The equipment can be used for routine evaluation of blood pressure, pulse, respiration, temperature, and for other physical and physiological conditions. In the intensive care unit, it is important to have built-in alarm systems that will warn the staff of critical changes in the patient's condition. Types of cardiac monitoring equipment include visual readouts of cardiac rhythms at the patient's bedside, supplemented by heart rate meters with audio and visual alarms, pacemakers with automatic or manual controls, and electrocardiograph recordings. At the nurses' station, there is usually a central panel that includes heart rate meters with audio and visual alarms.

Unlike telemonitoring equipment, bedside terminals involve nursing interaction. Nurses directly enter and retrieve patients' clinical data using bedside computer terminals. Data may include vital signs, lab results, and medications given. By utilizing bedside terminals, nurses are more productive and have more time to devote to patients and other nursing functions. In addition, by capturing data at the source or point of care, patient information is more accurate. It is ideal to integrate bedside terminals with the hospital's information system. This facilitates communication between nurses and other allied health professionals and results in more responsive patient care. The outcome of bedside terminals is an automated clinical record. This is a substitute for the traditional patient chart. A patient's clinical data is part of an integrated system that allows easy access to nurses, physicians, and allied health professionals.

NURSE STAFFING ISSUES

Because of labor force changes in most areas of the nation, a shortage of nurses as well as of other allied health professionals exists. Since the hospital is a labor-intensive industry, shortages can have a major impact on the operation of a hospital. Hospitals are meeting this challenging labor issue through the implementation of creative strategies. Some of these strategies include giving bonuses, using clinical career ladders to motivate and reward nurses involved in direct patient care, allowing nurses to budget for their unit, broadening job responsibility and autonomy, providing in-service training, and offering child day care services. Staffing issues will be present for many years because 1) the average age of a nurse in the United States is above 40, 2) for every eight nurses who leave the field, only five enter, and 3) the baby-boom population is aging and will be in increasing need of care (see Figure 10-4).

As mentioned earlier, the effect of the 2005 California law mandating a patient-to-nurse ratio of 5 to 1 will be interesting to observe. How many states are likely to follow this, and if they do, how acute will the nursing shortage become?

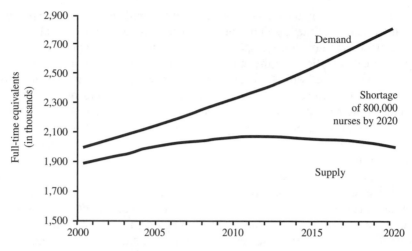

Figure 10-4 Forecast of total registered nurses: full-time equivalents vs. requirements, 2001-2020. *Source:* Bureau of Health Professionals, National Center for Health Workforce Analysis, *Projected Supply, Demand, and Shortages of Registered Nurses: 2000-2020*, released July 2002.

CHAPTER REVIEW

1. Name three educational paths to becoming an RN.
2. List three different types of nurses recognized by states.
3. What are two ways nursing staffs may be organized in a hospital?
4. Describe several types of special patient care units.
5. Describe four modes of nursing delivery.
6. What are three commonly used approaches to nurse scheduling?
7. How do nurses utilize bedside terminals?
8. Describe several methods hospitals use to cope with the nursing shortage.
9. You are the CEO of a 100-bed hospital and out of your 450 employees, 219 are nurses. You have an average daily census of 75 inpatients. Because of a flu epidemic, vacation leave, and a large bus wreck, you are experiencing both a spike in the census (you now have 94 patients) and have a shortage of nurses (you now have 191 nurses). What do you plan to do to have a full complement of nurses today and thus meet patient safety requirements?
10. Discuss the pros and cons of staffing the nursing department for "acuity of illness."

Part V
Tests and Results

Chapter 11

Key Ancillary Services

Key Terms

Ancillary	Medical imaging
Anesthesiologist	Nuclear medicine
Computerized tomography	Nurse anesthetist
(CT)	Pathologist
Freestanding imaging centers	Radiologist
Informed consent for surgery	Registered medical technologist
Laboratory information systems	Wilhelm Roentgen
Magnetic resonance imaging	Surgical specimens
(MRI)	Ultrasound

INTRODUCTION

The hospital's ancillary departments may also be called professional service departments. Literally, ancillary means assisting the physician in the diagnosis or treatment of the patient. An ancillary department is both a cost center (having expenses) and a revenue center (able to bill the patient for services) within the hospital, which requires, by regulation or third party urging, either that a physician directs the department or that a physician provides guidance and supervision over the department. In simple terms, what differentiates an ancillary service department from other hospital departments is that it is able to charge the patient directly, thereby generating revenue for the hospital, and it must be under the direction of a physician.

Ancillary departments are complex because their charge structure is different and consists of many individual tests. In addition, the departments have highly sophisticated equipment and a variety of well-trained technical staff. Another factor that makes these departments complex for management is physician compensation. There are varieties of ways in which the physicians who direct these departments may be reimbursed.

A typical large community hospital may have all of the ancillary departments discussed throughout this chapter, or it might have a selection of services such as a clinical laboratory services, radiology (or medical imaging), physical therapy, inhalation therapy, anesthesiology, dietary services, EKG (electrocardiography, heart station), and EEG (electroencephalography). The following sections provide some details and an analysis of three major ancillary departments—clinical laboratories, radiology, and anesthesiology—to illustrate the function of the organization and the way ancillary departments relate to physicians and patients.

THE CLINICAL LABORATORY DEPARTMENT

Clinical laboratories, another term for pathology departments, are of rather recent origin. Yet in their relatively short period of existence, they have undergone tremendous growth. Just before World War I, a typical hospital pathology department was small and ill equipped. Pathologists spent most of their time doing simple urinalyses, blood counts, and a few chemical determinations in bacteriology. Only a few surgical specimens (tissue removed by the physician during surgery) were examined, and only a few autopsies were performed. After World War I, the pathology and clinical laboratory departments began to grow. Physicians, having learned the value of pathology services from their war experiences, began to demand such services in civilian hospitals.

Between 1875 and 1900, the field of bacteriology rapidly grew. In fact, most of the known important pathogenic microorganisms were isolated in this period. However, it was several years before bacteriology became widely applied. It was not until 1937 that blood banking was used as a practical procedure in hospitals. Following World War II, additional growth occurred. New knowledge on how to expose health and disease problems proliferated. Diagnostic radioisotopes, exfoliative cytology, molecular diseases, practical virology, and fluorescent studies were introduced.

Clinical Laboratory Functions

A hospital's clinical laboratory has a number of functions, but its primary purpose is to provide information to assist physicians and other members of the health team in the diagnosis, prevention, and treatment of disease. The principal mission is accomplished by performing bacteriologic, biochemical, histologic, serologic, and cytologic tests in the laboratory.

The clinical laboratory is responsible for the blood bank as well. Blood banking as a regular service in hospitals is concerned with such blood procedures as cross matching, compatibility testing, and the procurement, preparation, and storage of blood prior to transfusion. Another major concern for the blood bank is screening for contaminated blood products. An additional responsibility for the clinical laboratory could be the operation of the hospital's morgue. Other related functions of the clinical laboratory depend on the size and complexity of the hospital; these can involve training programs and research.

One of the important ways a laboratory improves the quality of medicine is through its formal reports, especially on postmortem examinations and on examinations of tissues removed in surgical operations (surgical specimens).

The Tissue Committee serves as a classic quality control mechanism. Usually comprised of the pathologist and several surgeons, it reviews specimen reports to uncover surgeons that have undertaken unnecessary operations, e.g., a "hot appendix" is diagnosed but then after removal, the tissue is found by the pathologist to be quiet normal. If several of these operations occur, the surgeon performing the operations may be recommended for further training, recommended to be supervised by other physicians, or may even be suspended from the hospital staff.

Organization of the Clinical Laboratory

The department is organized under the leadership and directorship of a pathologist. This licensed physician specializes in the practice of pathology and is usually eligible for certification or is certified by the American Board of Pathology in either clinical or anatomical pathology, or perhaps both.

The department itself can be divided into two major sections—a clinical pathology division and an anatomical pathology section. The clinical laboratory and pathology services fall into two areas: 1) those performed directly by the pathologist and 2) those under the pathologist's responsibility and supervision but actually conducted by a medical technologist.

It is the pathologist's task to examine all surgical specimens (including those from autopsies, frozen sections, and tissue consultations). Under the pathologist's supervision, a medical technologist's functions may fall into these areas: 1) bacteriology; 2) biochemistry; 3) blood bank; 4) hematology; 5) tissue preparation; 6) organ banks, which some hospitals have for the storing of human organs and tissues used in transplant surgery (for example, corneas and kidneys); and 7) nuclear medicine and isotopes.

Some hospitals may contract with private laboratories outside the hospital known as reference labs for advanced testing.

Staffing of the Clinical Laboratory

The majority of employees in the clinical laboratories are usually registered medical technologists or medical laboratory technicians. A registered technologist must complete a bachelor's degree in an accredited college or university by taking specified science courses in a school of medical technology approved by the Council on Medical Education and the Hospitals of the American Medical Association. The technologist must then pass an examination given by the American Society of Clinical Pathologists (ASCP).

Other personnel working in the clinical laboratory include blood bank technologists, certified laboratory assistants, cytotechnologists, histotechnologists, and microbiologists.

There may be some nonregistered personnel working in the clinical laboratory, since there is a shortage of qualified personnel in certain parts of the country. From time to time, persons with PhD degrees in special science disciplines (such as chemistry) also work in the department.

The number of employees will vary with the workload in the department. Departments that are heavily involved in teaching or research or that handle outside requests will obviously employ more staff. A specific hospital staffing pattern can only be determined after an on-site analysis is conducted and knowledge of the specific workloads within the hospital is available.

As for the medical technologists themselves, there have been studies that suggest what the average workload for a technologist should be per year. These studies consider the types of tests and indicate the differences between hospitals that have a high, medium, or low volume. A staffing and workload analysis is critical when one determines how much space and equipment is needed to run a proper laboratory operation. Experience with improved techniques in automation suggests that a greater volume of work can be done in the same work area, depending on the clinical laboratory involved.

Location and Physical Facilities of the Clinical Laboratory

Laboratory facilities were at one time located either on the ground floor or on the first floor because the first floor offers easy accessibility to the outpatients who are sent to the laboratory. This has changed with the advent of conveniently located specimen drawing areas. It is not as important for inpatients to come to this area, since much of the laboratory's work (that is, collecting specimens) is done in the patient care units. In determining the overall size of the laboratory, it is important that consideration be given to each functional technical unit—that is, microbiology, chemistry, hematology, and pathology. Only after the size of each unit has been established can architectural layouts be properly constructed to fit into the complete program of the laboratory department. A square-foot-per-patient-bed ratio is not considered a completely adequate guide for determining the size of a laboratory. Any plans for a laboratory should be based on work volumes within specific ranges within the laboratory itself. For example, 40,000 to 75,000 laboratory tests equates to so many square feet of necessary laboratory space. Small hospitals (those with 20–40 beds) may have one laboratory. However, many larger hospitals could be expected to have laboratories that include separate work units for all technical sections—hematology, urinalysis, biochemistry, histology, serology, and bacteriology. Special support areas for glass washing and sterilizing are also available. The pathologist's office and the secretarial/reception area are in separate cubicles. Laboratory specimens may be received directly from the patient care units throughout the day and from specially located drawing stations in several parts of the hospital, such as the ED.

Clinical Laboratory Information Systems

It is essential that test results be placed in a report format and promptly and accurately provided to the physicians and health professionals who need to know the results. Traditionally, laboratories have manually handled record keeping and reports.

With the growing demand for laboratories to handle more patients and process their test results faster and more efficiently, many hospitals today use automated laboratory information systems. An automated system has the ability to provide quick test ordering, test tracking, and test result reporting. Laboratory data can be presented in a more orderly and timely manner. Physicians, nurses, medical technologists, and other allied health professionals have access to test results as soon as tests are completed. Other benefits include reduced reporting errors and improved legibility.

Automated information systems may also be used to gather statistics on physician ordering and to study certain susceptibilities in patients in order to optimize drug dosages as prescribed by physicians.

In addition to the benefits of increased speed and accuracy in reporting results, automated systems are also used to create anatomic pathology reports, to report on quality control, and to maintain inventory control records.

Laboratory Quality Review

In addition to JCAHO's quality review of hospitals (discussed in Chapter 24), the College of American Pathologists (CAP) has its own quality review program for laboratories. Quality in the laboratory not only includes accuracy and precision but also the quick reporting of results to patients. The CAP collects data about blood utilization and cost utilization, analyzes the lab's performance, and sends a report to the laboratory along with the aggregate performance of other labs. Hospitals are able to review lab performance with respect to turnaround time, reporting errors, and nosocomial infection rates and compare it with other laboratories.

Summary: The Clinical Laboratory

The clinical laboratory has become an essential factor in the care of patients within the hospital. Laboratory tests and examinations are growing rapidly in number and complexity. Since diagnosis and research in medical care are also extremely broad and intensive, the hospital pathologist becomes a critical element in the care of each patient. Because of automation, much of the laboratory testing is of routine nature and has been relegated to sophisticated equipment that can produce numerous tests in a brief period.

The pathologist is the spokesperson not only for this department, but also in a way is the conscience of the medical staff. The pathologist's crucial role on the tissue committee involves interpreting and guiding physicians' practices through laboratory procedures and tests. This department, and the pathologist in particular, are key elements in the hospital's quality improvement program.

THE IMAGING DEPARTMENT

If diagnosis is the cornerstone of modern medicine, the medical imaging department, which was once called the x-ray department, is the cornerstone of medical diagnosis. The field of radiology had its beginning on November 8, 1895, when Wilhelm Roentgen, an astute observer and professor of physics at the University of Wurzburg in Bavaria, discovered x-rays. News of the discovery traveled quickly. Within a matter of weeks, physicists and physicians throughout the world were producing x-rays of various types. They were quickly applied to the practice of medicine.

X-rays, when properly applied, permit a trained physician to recognize many medical conditions otherwise not diagnosable in a living patient. In addition, radiation beams carefully administered in sufficient doses have been found to be an effective treatment method for many diseases. These beams, emitted from x-ray tubes, gave birth to such devices as datatrons and cyclotrons, which are important in therapeutic radiology. This led to a separate discipline called radiation therapy, or radiotherapy. High-energy machines such as linear accelerators, employing high particle acceleration, are also used in radiotherapy. Considerable progress is being made toward further use of diagnostic and therapeutic radiation procedures.

Functions of the Imaging Department

The principal functions of the imaging (old term: radiology) department are to assist the physicians and other health team members in the diagnosis and therapy of a patient's disease with imaging, fluoroscopy, magnetism, radioisotopes, and ultrasound waves. (The term radiology no longer correctly fits since MRI machines use magnetism instead of radiation to produce images and, similarly, ultrasound machines use sound waves to produce images.)

A secondary mission of the radiology department is to engage in essential research for medical advancement and to participate in educational and in-service programs for hospital residents and the medical staff. Finally, the hospital might be involved in the training of radiological technologists and other imaging technical specialists.

There are several special procedures or diagnostic methods used in a modern hospital imaging department. Fluoroscopy is a means by which body structures are viewed by sending x-rays through the body part to be examined and then observing the shadows cast on a fluorescent (glowing) screen. Cineradiography is a means of converting the fluorescent screen images into radiographs or even into motion pictures. Stereoscopy is the method of taking two radiographs from slightly different angles, thereby allowing physicians to view the body structure in three dimensions.

Advances in imaging because of computerization have led to the utilization of high-tech methods in the imaging department. One of the first applications of x-rays and computers was computerized axial tomography (CAT or CT scan). In a CT scan, a carriage is rotated, allowing an imaging team to scan a narrow cross section of the body. Many such scans are taken—perhaps as many as 180—at very small distances from each other. These images are then collected and displayed with the use of a computer. While an x-ray can only scan a fractured or broken bone, a CT scan can also reveal infection and bleeding. Some computerized tomography utilizes three-dimensional imaging, capable of rotating images to give different views of various tissues.

While computerized tomography uses radiation to create an image, magnetic resonance imaging (MRI) can expose internal anatomy without using ionizing radiation. The patient lies in a machine that resembles a tunnel. Intensive magnetic force causes the protons found in the molecules of the body to spin and align. This proton movement gives off energy signals, which are measured by radio frequency and assembled into clear photographic images of cross sections of the body. The MRI is able to produce pictures that show changes in bone marrow and the stages of hemorrhage. Tumors, tendons, ligaments, and cartilage also show up more clearly in MRI, again using magnetism rather than radiation.

Both computerized axial tomography and magnetic resonance imaging can only show the structural makeup of tissue. There is a newer imaging method called positron emission tomography (PET) that is capable of providing three-dimensional metabolic and functional views of organs. The equipment used is a cyclotron. It generates radioisotopes to produce cross-sectional images of the body. PET is particularly valuable in the diagnosis of coronary artery disease as it allows cardiologists to study cardiac tissue without using invasive procedures like cardiac catheterization. In addition, PET has been utilized to diagnose stroke, brain tumors, epilepsy, Alzheimer's disease, and schizophrenia.

There is another imaging method called ultrasound that uses a Doppler technique to scan internal organs. It produces moving shadows on a display screen. Special probes are designed for specific anatomical regions, which enable rapid diagnosis of internal organs. Ultrasound has been widely used to visualize a fetus within a mother's womb. Fetal abnormalities can be detected, and the sex of the unborn child can usually be distinguished. Some ultrasound instruments have Doppler techniques capable of displaying blood flow and diagnosing cardiac problems.

Nuclear Medicine

In many hospitals, nuclear medicine may be part of the imaging department. Nuclear medicine procedures, like other imaging methods, are valuable techniques in diagnosis and treatment. However, nuclear medicine procedures give medical personnel the ability to assess tissue function as well as metabolism and blood flow. An imaging agent called a radiopharmaceutical is injected into a patient. Radiopharmaceuticals contain a small amount of a radioactive element that attaches itself to organs. The agent used is dependent on the specific organs under study. A camera records the radioactivity emitted by the organ and surrounding tissue, and a planar image is produced. Nuclear medicine has a technology similar to computerized tomography called single photon emission computed tomography (SPECT). Like CAT scans, SPECT produces cross sections of an organ. It can more accurately detect heart and brain abnormalities than other nuclear medicine procedures. SPECT also has growth potential in the evaluation of bone disorders and detecting tumors, trauma, and infection.

A recent advance in technology is the Gamma Knife. The patient can benefit from brain surgery using a focused gamma beam, called a Gamma Knife, without the cranium being opened.

Radiation Therapy

A type of ancillary service related to medical imaging is radiation therapy, which is a form of treatment used in the control of localized cancers. This service is generally found in larger hospitals and regional medical centers. Traditional imaging equipment uses x-rays or roentgen rays that are applied to electromagnetic, nonparticulate, ionizing radiation that is produced by manmade machines. In radiation therapy, radiations are either naturally occurring or artificially produced from radioactive elements. The equipment used may include a linear (electron) accelerator or a similar device called a betatron. This equipment generates high-energy radiations. Patients undergoing radiation therapy usually receive small doses several times a week for a period of 4 to 7 weeks. This service may be the responsibility of the hospital radiologist, but often there is a separate clinical department of radiation therapy headed by a physician trained in advanced physics.

The imaging department is also responsible for invasive procedures. There is a commonly used procedure called angiography, which is a technique using a contrast medium and injecting it into a patient's blood vessel, thereby allowing the blood supply (with the contrast medium) to reveal the structure and state of health of an organ.

Organization of the Imaging Department

In large hospitals, the imaging or radiology department may be organized into three separate sections: diagnostic radiology, therapeutic radiology, and nuclear medicine. In small hospitals, these may be arranged in one organization. The department is under the general direction and supervision of a competent radiologist, a graduate of a medical school who is licensed to practice in the state. This person is appointed as a member of the medical staff and should have considerable specialized training in radiology —diagnostic, therapeutic, or both—and be certified by the American Board of Radiology, which also certifies radiation therapists. Frequently the radiologist supervises the chief imaging technician. The radiologist is the clinical department head and, accordingly, has all the medical and administrative responsibilities that go with that position. In the larger context, the radiologist, as administrator of the department, is responsible to the administrator of the hospital; as a specialist concerned with the quality of care, the radiologist is responsible to the medical staff. Members of the medical staff send their patients to the department for diagnosis and treatment. The outpatient services account for approximately 50 percent of all the imaging work, including that from the emergency department. The various inpatient nursing units also send patients to the department for procedures during the working day.

Location and Physical Facilities of the Imaging Department

The imaging department, or at least a portion of it, should be located on the first floor of the hospital in order to be conveniently accessible to outpatients and inpatients scheduled for admission, and it should be near the emergency department for the convenience of the patient and trauma team. It is preferable to locate the imaging department close to elevators and adjoining the outpatient department. It is also best to locate the department in a wing of the hospital with the imaging rooms at the extreme end of the wing. In such a configuration, the traffic pattern through the department will be minimized and less shielding would be required due to the exterior walls around the imaging rooms.

A well-planned imaging diagnostic department will promote an efficient flow of service, thereby allowing patients to be scheduled properly and expediently with a minimum of movement and distance for both the imaging staff and the patients. The number of imaging machines to be installed in the unit will depend, of course, on the size of the hospital, the number of beds in the hospital, the volume of the emergency department, and the needs of the community that the hospital services.

Flexibility in the design of the department is important, particularly in a smaller hospital. It is a prerequisite for the handling of a potential increase in the workload and volume. If sufficient space is allocated to begin with, an increase in volume can be handled quite easily by adding additional staff members and installing another machine. When designing and planning an imaging department or reviewing whether an imaging department should be expanded, procedure standards for room utilization are extremely helpful. There may be individual variations due to the complexity of the examination mix; however, there are guidelines that can be used in determining the number of examination rooms necessary in the imaging area. Most often, statutes of the state regulating agency will influence the layout.

Staffing of the Imaging Department

The basic employee in the radiology department is the imaging technologist, or x-ray technician. There must be a sufficient number of these employees in the department to respond to the patients' needs. These technologists should be trained in imaging modalities and should be eligible for membership in the American Society of Radiologic Technologists. Technicians perform their work under the supervision of the radiologist and usually a chief technician. Two or three technicians will be required, depending on the workload (volume) and the value of the cases. Factors to be considered are the patients' status (whether or not they are ambulatory) and whether the technicians transport the patients themselves. Technologists must be additionally trained to operate the commonly used high-tech imaging methods, though most will find themselves specializing in one device such as CT or MR once they have learned the correct techniques.

FREESTANDING IMAGING CENTERS

Today, a growing number of hospitals are providing diagnostic and therapeutic radiological procedures in outpatient centers separate from the hospital. These centers are referred to as freestanding imaging centers. The advantages of freestanding imaging centers include better reimbursements for outpatient procedures than for inpatient procedures, a patient referral source for the hospital, and more convenience to the patient. Often these are joint ventures with physician staff members and unfortunately for the hospital, are sometimes completely physician owned.

Some hospitals are also involved in mobile diagnostic and therapeutic radiologic procedures. They offer radiological services in mobile vans as a way to take these services to patients at other hospitals or at work sites.

THE ANESTHESIOLOGY DEPARTMENT

The development of anesthesia began with the introduction of ether by Dr. William Morton, a Massachusetts dentist, in 1847. Unlike the development of anesthesia in Great Britain, the practice of anesthesia in the United States was not always a physician discipline. Though there were some surgeons who became interested in the problems of anesthesia, these represented a minority. It was not until the 1930s, when the study of the physiology of trauma in surgery began to unfold, that physicians became acutely interested in the discipline of anesthesiology.

Anesthesia received a great boost during World War II, when many of the physicians in the military, particularly in the army, were given training in anesthesia before being sent to the hospitals to work. Today anesthesiology is one of the largest specialty groups in the United States, with many members having the title of Fellow of the American College of Anesthesiologists. Until World War II, nurse anesthetists were the principle professionals involved in the administering of anesthesia. (While nurse anesthetists still practice in many hospitals, many hospitals now prefer to have Board Certified Anesthesiologists.)

A nurse anesthetist is a registered professional nurse who has been trained in the administration of anesthesia. The nurse anesthetist may also assist patients with respiratory or cardiopulmonary conditions. After completing education and certification, the individual may use the initials CRNA (Certified Registered Nurse Anesthetist) after his or her name.

Functions of the Anesthesiology Department

The anesthesiology department has four main functions: 1) to render a patient insensible to pain during a surgical procedure, 2) to control the patient's physiology during the procedure, 3) to follow the patient during the immediate postoperative period, and sometimes, 4) to operate an outpatient center for pain management. The anesthesia department is also responsible for providing local or block anesthesia in certain surgical procedures, such as childbirth.

Hospital administrators, nurses, physicians, and anesthesiologists all must be aware that patients going to surgery are required to sign certain permission slips (informed consent for surgery) prior to surgery. A patient must be informed about the surgical procedure and the liabilities and risks involved before signing the permit to undergo the procedure. It is also the anesthesiologist's responsibility to visit the patient prior to surgery. The patient should be informed about what anesthesia will be used, how it will be administered, and what that patient may feel.

Anesthesiologists also have a role in caring for critical or intensive care patients. They may function as primary care physicians, cooperate with primary care physicians, or act as consulting physicians. Anesthesiologists are involved with patients' dietary management and patients' problems regarding respiratory and circulatory insufficiency.

Organization of the Anesthesiology Department

Many hospitals have a separate department of anesthesiology. Those hospitals that do not have a separate department usually include anesthesia as a function of the department of surgery. Most often, the department of anesthesiology is headed by a physician who is trained in the medical discipline of anesthesia and is, as a rule, board certified. The department frequently has more than one physician anesthesiologist. It is quite common to have nurse anesthetists in the department. Both the physician specialist and the nurse anesthetist administer anesthesia. When a physician anesthesiologist is not available, for example, some rural hospitals may use nurse anesthetists exclusively to administer anesthesia. The responsibility for this department is then delegated to the chief of surgery or to another designated person. In such cases, the operating surgeon is responsible for the professional acts of the nurse anesthetists.

Location and Physical Facilities of the Anesthesiology Department

The anesthesiology department is usually near the hospital's operating suite. A typical layout for an operating room is shown in Figure 11-1.

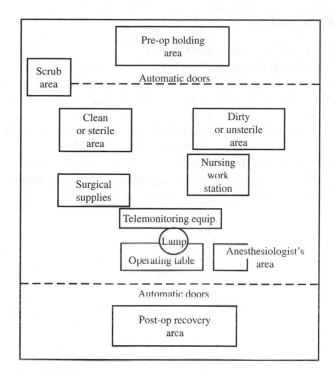

Figure 11-1 Floor plan for a typical operating room.

Staffing of the Anesthesiology Department

The precise number of physician anesthetists and nurse anesthetists employed in a given hospital will depend upon the number and types of surgical procedures and the number of obstetrical deliveries in the hospital. Personnel in the anesthesia department are required to be on call; this, of course, has an impact on staffing patterns. The nurse anesthetists, depending on the contractual arrangement between the anesthesiologist and the hospital, either work directly for the anesthesiologist or are hospital employees. In any event, the nurse anesthetists function under the technical supervision of the anesthesiologist.

CHAPTER REVIEW

1. How are ancillary departments defined?
2. What are some examples of ancillary departments?
3. What is the professional reviewing organization for the laboratory?
4. Why has the traditional name of the radiology department changed to imaging?
5. What is the difference between an anesthesiologist and a CRNA?
6. Discuss several major functions of the hospital pathologist.
7. Discuss other functions for anesthesiologists besides their role in surgery.
8. Why is it important to the quality improvement program that we send surgery specimens to the pathology department?

Chapter 12

Other Ancillary Services

Key Terms

Comprehensive outpatient
   rehabilitative facility (CORF)
Decentralized pharmacy
Electrocardiography
Electroencephalography
Floor stock

Formulary unit dose system
Narcotic drugs
Occupational therapist
Physical therapist
Pulmonary function studies
Ventilators

INTRODUCTION

Chapter 11 contained an overview of the laboratory, imaging, and anesthesia departments. Other critical ancillary services are respiratory therapy, EEG, the cardiac center, physical therapy, occupational therapy, speech therapy, and the pharmacy.

RESPIRATORY CARE DEPARTMENT

A discipline closely related to anesthesiology is respiratory therapy. The respiratory care field has developed rapidly under the sponsorship of such organizations as the American College of Physicians and the American Society of Anesthesiologists. In today's hospital, respiratory therapy is an extremely important facet in the diagnosis and treatment of certain categories of patients. The respiratory care department at one time was known as the inhalation therapy department. The older term referred to the treatment of patients with the use of oxygen and other inhalation therapies.

The respiratory care department embodies the therapeutic value of oxygen and other therapies together with pulmonary function studies (measuring a patient's lung capacity and output, this being especially useful in the diagnosis of smoking-related diseases and also in the field of sports medicine) and blood gas analysis. The department is involved in both diagnostic and therapeutic treatment of inpatients and outpatients. It is an important unit in the treatment and diagnosis of patients with pulmonary disease and certain cardiac ailments. It is responsible for administering breathing treatments such as bronchodilator therapies to patients, setting up equipment for oxygen administration, giving chest physiotherapy to patients, and managing the adequate functioning of ventilators. The respiratory department also participates in cardiac arrest codes by providing all the equipment and supplies needed to assist the patient with ventilation. Typically the respiratory therapist will "bag" the patient (breathing for the patient by using a mechanically assisted breathing device) freeing up the physician and remaining code team members to deliver chest compressions and drugs to the patient in cardiac arrest. All procedures given to the patients are performed by either a physician or a trained respiratory therapist. With the exception of emergencies, these procedures usually can be administered to the patient only under the prescribed written orders of a physician.

ELECTROENCEPHALOGRAPHY

One of the more specialized ancillary services in hospitals is the electroencephalography (EEG) testing service. This is generally part of the neurosurgery or neurology section of the hospital or medical staff. This service is an indispensable tool for solving neurosurgical or neurological problems. The EEG test measures the electrical brain activity of the patient. It is frequently used when patients have suffered serious head injuries; in such circumstances, an EEG test can be essential to saving the life of the patient. EEG testing was formerly used primarily for the diagnosis of seizures and the detection of tumors. However, in recent years, EEG tests have been utilized in analyzing many problems, from fainting and mild headaches to epileptic disorders and severe trauma from a head injury. The test is conducted by highly trained technicians upon a physician's order. The EEG test must be conducted in a room where extraneous noise cannot be picked up. If the room is not perfectly situated, certain objects will appear on the EEG readout and render it useless. The EEG laboratory does not have high volume like laboratory and imaging do. Frequently, however, EEG lab technicians are on 24-hour call for emergency situations. The EEG tests are used in determining both the first signs of life and the last signs of life coming from the brain.

There are hybrids of EEG techniques that include studies of when the patient is awake or asleep. Sleep EEGs are particularly important in the study of different types of epilepsy. EEG tests are frequently used in combination with CT scanners to assist physicians in giving diagnoses that are more complete.

The diagnostic role of electroencephalography has been expanded to include a therapeutic one. This has been illustrated by employing EEGs in sleep disorder clinics to treat patients with problems such as sleep apnea.

THE CARDIAC CENTER

Diagnostic services for the heart are usually provided in the area of the hospital commonly referred to as the cardiac center. One of the core products of this "heart station" is electrocardiography (EKG).

The EKG is used most frequently on patients with cardiac disease, including those with complications, and suspected cardiac disease. It is also useful as a chest baseline test prior to surgery. If an electrocardiogram is abnormal, detailed information regarding the diagnosis and management of the patient is provided; this makes the course of the patient's treatment much more reliable and scientific. An electrocardiogram is taken with special equipment to produce an electrocardiograph. The basic EKG machine is a table-type apparatus on wheels that is rolled to the inpatient's bedside and is operated by skilled technicians.

The interpreter of the cardiogram is usually a cardiologist or an internist who is skilled in reading electrocardiogram tracings. The technician must be trained to take multilead tracings, that is, tracings from the 12 leads that are normally attached to the patient to obtain a routine electrocardiogram.

Hospitals may use a three-channel EKG cart with computerized printout attachments as part of their equipment. In this arrangement, the technician goes to the patient's bedside with an electrocardiograph cart that has a telephone receiver attached. The tracings are sent electronically to be read, relayed to a computer that interprets it as an unconfirmed electrocardiograph; it is unconfirmed because the computer, not a cardiologist, has read it. A hospital cardiologist then performs an over-read of the computerized interpretation printout and confirms it. The physician who reads the printout signs it as if the technician in the hospital had taken a paper tracing and hand-carried it to the physician for reading and interpretation. The two advantages of the shared computerized electrocardiogram system are: 1) it offers a high degree of consistency and quality and 2) it provides rapid feedback on the readings.

Though the basic electrocardiogram is the most common service in hospitals, there are variations of electrocardiograph tracings that are done for different purposes to determine special diagnostic problems. For example, stress testing or treadmill exercise testing is a procedure in which a patient is placed under severe stress and the patient's heart impulses are then interpreted in those conditions. Hospitals use echoencephalography and Holter monitoring, procedures in which a patient wears a tracing or monitoring device while active for a period of hours; tracings are then made and interpreted through a computer reading.

Nuclear medicine procedures such as a multigated acquisition (MUGA) wall motion study and thallium single photon-emission computed tomography (SPECT) and planar tests are also used to evaluate patients with coronary artery disease, chest pain, and questionable EKG and stress tests. Other diagnostic testing provided by the cardiac center includes echocardiography, Doppler modalities, and peripheral vascular studies. Pacemaker insertion and evaluation can also be located in the cardiac center.

REHABILITATIVE MEDICINE—PHYSICAL THERAPY, OCCUPATIONAL THERAPY, AND SPEECH THERAPY

The discipline of physical medicine and rehabilitation, conducted by a specialist known as a physiatrist (physical medicine doctor) is a medical specialty concerned with the diagnosis and treatment of certain musculoskeletal defects and neuromuscular diseases and problems. Physical medicine began to emerge during World War I when the Army was involved in vocational guidance and training programs for the disabled. However, it was not until some time following World War II that the specialty became well known and formal training programs became more available.

The original 3-year residency in physical medicine and rehabilitation was established at the Mayo Clinic. Today, there are a growing number of hospitals specializing in complete physical medicine and rehabilitation services. A physical medicine department is headed by a physician whose special interests lie in physical medicine, sports medicine, and rehabilitation. The financial arrangements between the physiatrist and the hospital management are usually on a simplified salaried or fee-for-service basis. Fee-for-service billing is a method whereby a physician bills the patient or third party for each physician service given.

Areas of rehabilitative medicine include physical therapy (PT), occupational therapy (OT), and speech therapy. Physical therapy is prescribed by a physician and the referred patient is evaluated and treated by the physical therapist staff of the hospital. These professionals have earned a bachelor's, master's, or doctoral degree in physical therapy, or they have a postbaccalaureate certificate of training. Physical therapists are licensed by each state, which usually requires an MS.

Those with a BS are usually physical therapist assistants (PTAs). The therapist uses light, heat, water, electricity, ultrasound, and physical/mechanical force to treat the patient's illness or pain.

Although physical facilities vary widely, hospitals usually have a large room or gymnasium for physical therapy. In this area, there is sufficient space for patient cubicles, dressing rooms, toilets, showers, and a range of physical therapy equipment. This equipment may include diathermy units, ultrasound devices, gym mats, Hubbard tanks, parallel walking bars, ultraviolet lamps, whirlpool baths, exercising steps, progressive resistance apparatus, and treatment tables.

Hospitals may also offer occupational therapy services under the direction of a physician. The occupational therapist is involved in treating physical disability and in teaching the patient compensatory techniques to perform daily activities, frequently with the assistance of self-help aids. The occupational therapist is also involved in perceptual testing and training. The therapist is guided by the physician when creating certain educational and functional activities to help patients. Like the physical therapist, the occupational therapist has earned a master's degree in occupational therapy; occupational therapy assistants may be licensed with a BS.

Finally, speech therapy has become more common in community hospitals. This therapeutic discipline uses speech therapists and physicians to correct a patient's speech defect or to reeducate the patient who may have lost the ability to speak due to disease, accident, or stroke. Often, speech therapists are involved in emphasizing methods to correct speech and language debilities with the objective of bringing patients back as close as possible to normal speech functions. The speech therapist has a master's or doctoral degree and has been registered with the state.

Medicare has approved the concept of outpatient rehabilitative medicine by permitting hospitals to set up comprehensive outpatient rehabilitation facilities (CORFs). A CORF is a nonresidential facility that is established to provide diagnostic, therapeutic, and restorative services. Services are provided at a single, fixed location, by or under the supervision of a physician. The services include physical therapy, occupational therapy, and speech therapy, as well as supportive service in psychology, social services, and orthotics/prosthetics.

THE PHARMACY

The hospital pharmacy may have the role of dispensing and compounding drugs and other diagnostic and therapeutic chemical substances that are used in the hospital. In very small hospitals there might not be a regular pharmacy department;

the hospital may instead purchase items from a local pharmacist and maintain only a limited supply under supervised security. In most hospitals, a full-time pharmacist is available, sometimes with several assistants. Currently, with pharmacists in short supply, many hospitals contract with an outside pharmacy company to supply personnel and manage the department.

Some hospitals have a decentralized pharmacy system with one main pharmacy and satellite pharmacies on each nursing unit of the hospital. Very modern hospitals have robots that deliver medications from the central pharmacy to patient rooms for dispensing by the nursing staff.

Some hospitals also operate outpatient pharmacies. The pharmacy might sell items to the public in addition to the patients, but this practice is generally discouraged and varies according to state law.

Whether the pharmacy department compounds certain solutions or drugs depends on hospital policy. For quality and financial reasons, most hospitals prefer to purchase drugs and solutions already made, whether for injections or intravenous administration.

The head pharmacist must be licensed and must have completed a 5-year program in an accredited school of pharmacy. Some pharmacists pursue a doctor of pharmacy degree (PharmD). Pharmacy technicians function to assist the pharmacist in prepackaging drugs, controlling inventory, distributing floor stock items, and assisting in activities not requiring professional judgment. Pharmacy technicians may be trained on the job or in a hospital-based program.

Pharmacy and Therapeutics Committee

The pharmacy and therapeutics committee functions as a liaison between the pharmacy and medical staff with the role of overseeing the medical aspects of the hospital's pharmacy activities. Members usually include physicians, a pharmacist, a nurse, and an administrator. Though the pharmacy and therapeutics committee recommends the standard drugs to be dispensed in the hospital, it is the pharmacist's responsibility in the vast majority of hospitals to select the brand or supplier of drug dispensed for all medication orders and prescriptions, unless a specific notation to the contrary is made by the prescriber.

A key duty of the pharmacy and the therapeutics committee is to develop a formulary of acceptable drugs. The formulary contains a list of drugs, usually by generic names, approved by the medical staff and available for use within the hospital. Recommended dosages, contraindications, warnings, and pharmacology are described in the formulary. Other functions of the committee include educating the medical staff when new drugs are introduced, reviewing drug reactions and studies, participating in quality improvement, and establishing cost-effective drug therapy.

Drug Distribution System

Once received in the hospital or pharmacy, drugs and supplies are distributed primarily to the nursing units. Inpatients receive the majority of drugs dispensed by the pharmacy. Generally, drugs fall into one of three categories:

1. Items sent to the nursing units for floor stock inventory. These are items regularly stored in the unit and not charged to patients directly. Examples of such nonchargeable items are rubbing compounds, antiseptics for wounds, and bandages.
2. Patient-chargeable stock items kept in the nursing unit. These include disposable enema packs and other disposable external preparations.
3. Common prescription drugs that are dispensed and charged only upon receipt of a prescription by a physician. This category of prescription drugs represents the vast majority of drugs used and represents the greatest cost in the pharmacy.

A common method of dispensing medication to patients is the unit dose system. The pharmacy either packages the medication or purchases prepackaged medications in specific dosages. The latter method allows for better control and less waste of the drug; on the other hand, this method carries the additional cost of packaging the drugs. Under the unit dose system, a 24-hour supply of medications is dispensed to each nursing unit. The medications are kept in patient drawers in the nursing unit's medication cart. The drawers are combined into cassettes, and cassettes are exchanged by the pharmacy at a designated time every day. The unit dose system offers greater convenience to the hospital pharmacist, nurses, and patients. With this system, there is increased efficiency of operations, and preparation and distribution errors are reduced.

The pharmacy department is also responsible for the preparation and distribution of intravenous fluid (IV) solutions or parenteral feeding products like nutritional substances and chemotherapeutic agents. The timing of preparation and delivery is crucial, since some solutions are stable for only a given time. A sterile environment is necessary for drug preparation; therefore, laminar flow hoods are needed for the pharmacy department preparing such solutions.

Control of Narcotics and Barbiturates

The hospital must exercise strict control over the dispensing of narcotics and barbiturates. These drugs must be kept under security both in the pharmacy (usually in a large safe) and in the nursing units (usually in very limited doses). Thorough and adequate records must be kept on narcotics and barbiturates. At the

Part VI

Behind the Scenes— The Support Services

IN GENERAL, WHAT ARE *SUPPORT* SERVICES?

Hospital support services may be defined as those hospital departments or cost centers that do not provide direct medical tests for patients, but in general support the hospital's mission. These services do not normally generate patient revenue and are not under the professional direction of a physician as required by JCAHO. There are three types of support services in a hospital: patient support service departments, facilities support service departments, and administrative support service departments. Patient support services may have direct patient contact and include the following areas or departments: dietary, social services, pastoral care, patient escort, and patient ombudsman/patient representative services. The facilities support services include the traditional plant operation services such as environment (housekeeping) services, engineering/maintenance, the physical plant, and clinical (biomedical) engineering department. The administrative support services are those nonpatient care departments that directly support the administrative mission of the hospital and include materials management, human resources, volunteers, and telecommunications departments. Chapters 13 through 15 will focus on support services.

Chapter 13

Patient Support Services

Key Terms

American Dietetic Association	Patient menus
Chaplain	Patient representa-
Contract services	tive
Convenience food	Patient transportation
Dietician	Special diets
Discharge planning	Social worker

DIETARY DEPARTMENT

Probably no department in the hospital reaches more patients, hospital staff, and visitors than the dietary department. If the food service is efficient and effective, it usually receives only faint praise from patients and personnel. If the food service is perceived to be lacking in quality, criticisms abound. Complaining patients often say, "For what I am paying for this room, you would think that the food would be better"; "It should be hot"; or "I could have it when I want it if I were in a hotel." These comments speak to the crucial public relations aspect of the dietary department.

In earlier times, the preparation and delivery of food were under the auspices of the nursing department, the head housekeeper, or the chief cook. The housekeeping department underwent an evolution and the dietary department started to take on a separate entity—food services were removed from the nursing department. Developments in the world of nutrition and dietetics had an impact on the formation of special dietary departments. The medical profession began to study the role of proper diet and nutrition as an aid to maintaining good health. A second development was the evolution of the dietetics into a professional field. The American Dietetic Association, the professional group of those practicing in the dietary field, has given emphasis to the sophisticated training of dieticians. Dieticians today usually have earned a bachelor's degree and sometimes a master's degree and then spend a year in an internship before earning a registered dietician (RD) degree, which many states (and JCAHO) require before hospital employment.

The dietary department has a role in the therapeutic care of patients as well as in providing standard food menus for patients and staff. Dieticians plan and direct food and meal service and educate patients in proper nutrition.

Patient Menus

It is the dietician's responsibility to plan menus for patients and staff. The hospital dietician must have sound technical knowledge about foods as well as sufficient imagination to group foods attractively for meals. Dieticians must be sensitive to the psychological impact that food can have on the well-being of patients. Contemporary hospitals find themselves catering to the patient's wants, as well as to their nutritional needs. They offer a selection of meats, vegetables, and desserts, including out-of-season products and hothouse fruits. Many hospitals offer gourmet menus.

Dieticians prefer 2- or 3-week schedules in preparing their menus. Basic outlines are used and daily adjustments are made to handle special diet needs. The selective menu (allowing patients to have more than one food choice) in hospitals has gained wide acceptance and use. As might be expected, the selective menu is easier to implement in larger hospitals. Menus are modified by having the dietician regularly visit patients to determine their requests. The public relations aspect of a dietician's visit cannot be underestimated. Improving the nutritional services by reducing patient complaints and making the patients feel they are special, as they should be, is a crucial part of the hospital dietician's role.

Special Diets

There is an increasing use of special diets for hospital patients. This has occurred because of advances in diet therapy and a greater understanding of nutrition. Special diets are actually based on physicians' therapeutic orders that are placed in the patient's medical records. A physician, in consultation with the dietician, will recommend a specific diet based on a patient's condition. Special diets for patients are prepared under the direct supervision of a responsible dietician or nutritionist. Since the variety of food may be greatly reduced, it poses a real psychological challenge for the dietician to make the special tray attractive. Some examples of special diets are low sodium, low cholesterol, high fiber, restricted calorie, diabetic, clear fluids, full liquids, and pureed food.

Types of Food Service

Because of the increasing pressure on hospital management to contain costs but still to meet the demands and requests of patients and with the changing of state-of-the-art food service, hospitals have explored a variety of methods to produce and deliver high-quality meals. There are at least four systems in the preparation and delivery of food in hospitals: conventional, convenience food, cook–chill, and the frozen ready (cook–freeze) system. Food service experts describe the four systems as follows:

The *conventional* system uses a menu prepared daily from basic ingredients with preparation, assembly, and finishing, completed on the premises.

The *convenience food* system uses menu items that largely have been commercially prepared off premises and then have been frozen and/or freeze-dried in a form that can be easily prepared on site without the need for anything more complex than simple heating. An example of this type of item is the preplated hospital special-diet meal similar to the frozen TV dinner.

The *cook–chill* system makes use of on-site prepared products that are not necessarily utilized the day of preparation; they are flash-chilled, stored in the chill state (about 35 degrees F), and reheated immediately before service.

The *frozen ready (cook–freeze)* food primarily uses a menu that is mass-produced on site, frozen, and stored in a form that requires only thawing and reheating before service.

A hospital may use more than one system by selecting a combination of these four systems for its particular production system. Selection among the four systems is left to the dietician, food service manager, and hospital administration. The costs—operating cost per meal and annual cost per meal—may vary. The food costs in the convenience system are apt to be higher, and in the conventional system, lower.

Depending on the method of food production that the hospital selects, tray service to patients will vary. Essentially, there are two basic systems of tray service: centralized and decentralized. Many hospitals have modifications of each of these systems due to the physical layout of the hospital. The bulk food delivery system is really a hybrid of the centralized and decentralized systems.

Centralized systems are used by many hospitals because they provide greater efficiency, economy, and supervision, as well as efficient utilization of personnel time. Patient trays are centrally prepared and checked under central supervision along a conveyor belt, somewhat like an assembly line in the automobile industry.

The decentralized system is the oldest method of serving food. In a decentralized system, food is prepared and placed on the patients' trays in substations of patient care units. This is less efficient than the centralized system. Because each patient care unit needs a separate kitchen for the distribution of food, capital costs are increased. A weak link in the centralized food system may be in getting the tray to the patient's bedside. Since trays are brought to patient care units in large carts, food temperature may change in transit. New insulation trays can offset this; many have a heated pellet system housed in the tray to keep hot food hot.

Physical Facilities

Physical facilities of the food preparation area involve more than just a kitchen. The dietary area must have a method of receiving food products. For that reason, a receiving area and platform and an administrative area are necessary. In addition, once food is on the premises, it is important to see that there is clean and appropriate storage. There should be a central storage area, for both dry storage and refrigeration storage. Additionally, food production areas must be close to storage areas to reduce labor costs and the cost of transporting food to the area. In the food preparation area, there are cooking and baking facilities; numerous broilers, fryers, and ovens should be available. A dishwashing area should also be included.

Cafeteria Services

The hospital cafeteria, which provides cafeteria service for hospital staff, medical staff, visitors, and even ambulatory hospital patients, is usually within the jurisdiction of the dietary department. It is frequently near the food preparation area, so that service elevators or dumbwaiters can aid in transporting food from the food preparation section to the cafeteria. Two elements in the cafeteria are serving lines and the dining area.

At one time, hospital cafeterias essentially offered subsidized food as a fringe benefit; this allowed hospitals to rationalize lower salaries. As hospital employees' salaries have become more competitive, hospital cafeteria prices have also risen. Cafeteria services also have expanded. In addition to serving three hot and cold meals a day, many cafeterias have sandwich grills and snack services. Some hospitals contract out to fast-food companies to provide meals to employees and visitors.

Vending Services

Many times hospitals supplement their hospital cafeteria with food and beverage vending machines. It is frequently the dietary department's responsibility to oversee the hospital's vending operations. Usually these vending services are contracted out, but some hospitals do provide their own vending services. These provide food and snacks to employees and visitors who might be in the facility 24 hours a day.

Catering Services

The dietary department is responsible for catering services. Typically, catering services are for the administration, medical staff, and hospital functions such as community meetings and volunteer affairs. Although these services are labor intensive, they can create positive public relations for the dietary department and the hospital.

Contract Food Services

As hospitals continue to explore different methods of delivering and preparing food, they have also been exploring dietary department contract services.

An increasing number of hospitals engage outside management for their dietary and food areas, usually relying upon commercial companies for this purpose. The results range from quite satisfactory to unsatisfactory. There are pros and cons to hospital food-management contract services. Some of the advantages of having an outside contracting service include the use of highly specialized, trained personnel from an outside source, thereby reducing the need for hospital personnel and the recruitment of such specialists. Further, the outside management group may reduce costs through improved methods and efficiency. The byproduct of this may be fewer personnel and less food preparation equipment in the dietary area, depending on the method of food service selected. This could create space in the hospital and allow room for other departments. Any hospital using an outside food service firm should periodically review its performance.

Outside contractors would list as their advantages higher productivity, outstanding supervision, increased presentation skills, and the provision of advanced equipment and products. Outside contractors would then bring more flexibility to the hospital's changing environment. Nevertheless, there are advantages for the hospital to maintain its own in-house services. One advantage is loyalty from paid employees. Moreover, hospitals have found that with full-time employees of the hospital, certain scheduling flexibility may be achieved. In addition, a spirit of teamwork is generated by having the hospital use its own dietary department and by having its dietary employees work with other departments. Hospitals would also argue that having all the employees on the hospital's payroll enhances security. Proprietary food companies have a stake in offering their services at competitive prices and most demonstrate efficiency and effectiveness.

Expanded Food Service Programs

Hospitals have been expanding food service programs beyond traditional patient and employee services. New business lines have been created in response to underutilized services in the dietary department and a desire to generate revenue. Some examples of new food service programs are meals for the homebound, frozen dinners for local and regional markets, take-out delis, Sunday brunches for the public, bakeries, off-campus catering, and meals for nursing home residents.

SOCIAL SERVICES DEPARTMENT

Dr. Malcolm MacEachern, who is recognized as one of the early leaders in hospital administration, noted in his classic textbook, *Hospital Organization and Management,* that the 19th century British hospital had the equivalent of our social worker, who was called an "almoner." According to MacEachern, the almoner was the individual who represented the community that dispensed alms. The almoner's chief duty was to prevent abuse of charity. The almoner was also involved in hospital social programs. MacEachern traced this individual from the moralistic almoners of the Middle Ages, noting that the 19th century British counterpart had very little of the true spirit of charity. Apparently, the almoner's chief objective was offering aid but with the expenditure of as little money as possible. Whatever the merits of the 19th century almoner, this job appears to have been the forerunner of the present-day social worker's job in the hospital.

One of the United States' first organized social service departments in a hospital was formed by Dr. Richard C. Cabot at the Massachusetts General Hospital in 1905. At that time, a social worker was a fresh way to complement the efforts of physicians in delivering better medical care. Dr. Cabot's projected role for the newly formed profession was to search out and then report to the patient's physician various domestic and social conditions influencing the patient, and to form links between the hospital, other institutions, and the patient.

Qualifications of a Medical Social Worker

Social workers are educated individuals. Specifically, they must have graduated from a baccalaureate program or master's program; they are required by the state to be licensed. The American Association of Medical Social Workers has set forth the qualifications of training and eligibility for membership in that organization.

Functions of the Medical Social Worker

The modern-day hospital can expect the social service department to make at least six specific contributions to the mission of the hospital:

1. To aid the health team to understand the social, economic, and emotional factors that affect the patient's illness, treatment, and recovery
2. To aid the patient, the patient's family, and the hospital staff to understand these factors and to make constructive use of resources in the medical care system; this is a key part of efficient discharge planning
3. To promote the well-being of the patient and improve the patient's family's morale by working with the family and the patient
4. To improve the mission of the hospital by becoming involved in hospital education and activities with the hospital staff and members of the outside community
5. To offer better patient care by making various services, including those outside the hospital, available to the patient
6. To improve the utilization of the community's resources and to affect these resources in order to aid patient and family needs when the patient leaves the hospital

The social service department may also offer adoption assistance, information concerning community resources and support groups, home care services, assistance in acquiring durable medical equipment, and referrals to placement facilities, e.g., nursing homes. An important point is that if social service is to be effective, it must be directly related to communication with the physician and the patient.

A New Role for the Medical Social Worker

The social worker has taken on an important role in aiding the process of quality improvement. Working with the boundaries of the quality improvement program, social workers can make an important contribution in the area of discharge planning. JCAHO recommends that the social service department have a written policy and procedure for discharge planning. Discharge planning is the organized, centralized system to ensure that each hospitalized patient has a planned program to provide needed continuing care and the follow-up that he or she requires. Physicians, nurses, and administrators frequently rely on the social worker's assistance in arranging programs to enable patients to receive continuing care after they leave the hospital environment.

In order for discharge planning to be effective, it should begin at the time a patient is admitted to the hospital. A crucial aspect of discharge planning is the location of placement facilities such as long-term care and rehabilitation facilities for patients who are unable to go home following their hospitalization. This is a challenging task for the social worker. The social worker directly influences not only the patient's well-being, but also the cost effectiveness and efficiency of the hospital's operations. If the patient is not moved into a placement facility, the hospital could waste resources on further treatment. The social worker in the hospital environment has become an important asset of administration and the financial manager in saving the hospital money.

The medical social service department may yield intangible benefits. Though unmeasured in dollars, these benefits are reflected in the comments of the patients that social workers serve, as well as those of their families. Hospitals have found that medical social service departments have become an indispensable component in the hospital organization. Physicians frequently add their praise for the social worker, indicating their contribution to the rapid rehabilitation of patients.

Psychiatric Social Worker

There is a specialized role for social workers who work with patients who have emotional and mental as well as social and personal problems. Psychiatric social workers assist psychiatrists in diagnosis and treatment, help the patient's family to adjust, and engage in discharge planning activities. They are commonly experts in understanding community resources that a patient can turn to upon discharge.

PASTORAL CARE SERVICES

Chaplains and members of religious orders (e.g., nuns), function in the hospital as active listeners for patients and patients' families and as providers of non-secular support, especially in the ED and after surgery. The hospital chaplain engages in crisis intervention and stress management by helping the patient to discover and use his or her own spiritual strength and faith. Chaplains frequently act as intermediaries between the patient, the family, and the physician. Some chaplains take part in interdisciplinary staff meetings, read patients' clinical charts, and write notes in patients' medical records. They also can be key members of the hospital's bioethics committee.

PATIENT TRANSPORTATION SERVICES

The patient transport department provides transportation either by wheelchair or stretcher to patients who need to travel to various hospital areas for diagnostic and therapeutic procedures. A patient transporter may also assist the nursing staff in lifting patients out of and into their beds. Besides this physical contact, a patient transporter may socially interact with patients. Hospitals might have a centralized patient transportation service, depending on the hospital's auxiliary unit, or they might have decentralized services whereby individual hospital departments are responsible for providing their own patient transportation. Additionally, there are computer software programs that allow for scheduling quick and efficient patient transport in larger or complex hospitals.

THE PATIENT REPRESENTATIVE

Patient representative programs evolved in the late 1950s to ensure that patients were treated with dignity. In 1971, the Association of Patient Service Representatives was founded, and in 1972, the Society of Patient Representatives was recognized. Today, patient representative programs are common among hospitals.

Patient representatives function as liaisons among the patient, the family, and the complex health care and hospital system. Representatives are listeners, communicators, and facilitators. Duties of representatives include alleviating patients' anxieties, explaining hospital policies, investigating patient complaints, and sometimes attending to patients' emotional needs. Patient representatives also work closely with physicians, nurses, social workers, clergy, and risk managers in order to increase patient satisfaction and work toward a positive public image for the hospital. These workers often explain advanced directives and durable health care power of attorney forms to patients.

CHAPTER REVIEW

1. What several departments are involved in patient support services?
2. Describe four types of systems used to prepare and deliver foods in hospitals.
3. Describe two basic types of food services.
4. Why are vending services important in a hospital?
5. Discuss the pros and cons of a contract dietary food service.
6. What is the mission of a social worker?
7. What is the role of pastoral care services?
8. What is the role of a patient representative?
9. What is the role of the patient escort? Why is customer service training so important?

Chapter 14

Facilities Support Services

INTRODUCTION

This chapter will focus on those departments which support the medical center—the departments of 1) environmental services, 2) laundry, 3) mainte nance, 4) plant engineering, 5) parking, 6) security, 7) safety and disaster plan ning, and 8) biomedical engineering.

ENVIRONMENTAL SERVICES DEPARTMENT

Not long ago, environmental services, referred to as housekeeping services, were the responsibility of the nursing service department. As nurses increased their medical training and their duties shifted, a need arose for supporting the environmental department; thus, the creation of a separate functional area of environmental services. The department has two principal functions: to keep the hospital clean and to control the linen supply.

Keeping a hospital clean is challenging. Part of the problem is that a hospital is an active place, open 24 hours a day, every day of the year. High traffic areas need special attention to prevent a negative image of the entire hospital and to contain infections.

There is more to cleaning a hospital than simply making sure that each room and floor are cleaned properly—*why* cleaning is done is just as important as *what* is done. Cleanliness for hospital patients, visitors, and the medical staff has several side effects: it creates a positive public relations image; it has a psychological effect on patients and their visitors; the hospital seems to be well organized, and most importantly, a clean environment can reduce the probability of infection.

Staffing

The environmental services department is a labor-intensive department. It uses modern, up-to-date equipment, but the job of cleaning patient rooms, corridors, offices, and lobbies of the hospital falls to the labor force, made up primarily of sanitary specialists. The administrative head of the department is the executive housekeeper, chief housekeeper, or director of housekeeping. The housekeeping organization is conventional, in that it is based on a hierarchical principle with the chief housekeeper at the top, just above one or two assistants (supervisors), and followed by sanitary specialists.

Rank among the sanitary specialists is based on a traditional division of labor derived from historical job descriptions. Some are assigned light cleaning, dusting, and mopping of floors. Others do heavy housekeeping and furniture moving. These people are the front line of the environmental services department and are generally assigned to divisions, sections, or units in the hospital. A nursing unit can have one regularly assigned person with additional staff working the evening shift or on weekends. These key people have an impact on patients in several ways. The results of their work (that is, a clean nursing unit or patient bedroom) have both a public relations and psychological effect. The sanitary specialists' approach, professionalism, attitude, and personality directly affect each patient, since they come in daily contact with patients while cleaning their rooms. A cheerful, well-informed, polite employee, the product of a good guest relations program, can add much to the total image of the hospital.

Infectious and Hazardous Waste Removal

Today's hospital treats every patient with the concept of universal precautions, which recognizes that all patients have the potential of spreading HIV, hepatitis A, B, and C, etc. Believing every patient to be infectious, the housekeeping department must properly disinfect the patient's room and remove infectious, hazardous wastes. The department interfaces directly with the infection control committee's policies on disinfecting a given area or room, always using special bacterial solutions and certain misting or other techniques that have proven effective in disinfecting accommodations. Infectious wastes are always placed in specially marked red bags and double bagged. Incineration is the most efficient and cost effective method to dispose of infectious wastes, though legal and acceptable waste removal varies from state to state. Housekeepers must always wear gloves and watch for discarded needles in trash cans. Needle sticks can be life threatening due to infections.

The removal of hazardous wastes such as chemotherapy drugs and radioactive materials (radionuclides used in the imaging department) are regulated by local, state, and federal agencies. Many state laws concerning hazardous waste follow federal Environmental Protection Agency (EPA) regulations. The environmental services department must keep informed of changes in regulations. Hospitals may have on-site removal mechanisms such as incinerators, or they may contract with outside firms to provide waste removal services. The hospital, as creator of hazardous and infectious wastes (tissue removed during surgery, discarded blood products, patient specimens), is usually liable for safe and effective removal of these products.

HOSPITAL LAUNDRY

Hospitals often have their own hospital laundry, operated on the hospital grounds or in the hospital itself, or they may contract out laundry services. A typical hospital laundry will have areas set aside for receiving and sorting soiled linen. Other functional areas of the laundry are the washing room and the clean linen processing room, which has large tables for sorting, tumblers for drying, and machines for pressing. Besides the linen processing room, the laundry will also have a clean linen and pack preparation room where the clean linen is put on shelves for storage or placed directly into the decentralized linen carts. Administrators and laundry managers are continually seeking improved auto mated equipment to save time.

The head of the laundry department is the laundry manager. The laundry manager must possess skills in dealing with people and should understand laundry equipment and the technical aspects of laundering through proper solutions and washing formulas. The exact number of personnel required to operate a hospital laundry will vary with the number of beds in the hospital. If the laundry is responsible for retrieving soiled linens, distributing the linens, and packing certain sterile instruments, the number of personnel will increase.

The quantity of laundry needed must be determined. The usual standard is to have six complete sets of linen for each occupied bed. According to government studies, the six sets would be used as follows: one set on the patient's bed, one set en route to the laundry, one set being processed in the laundry, one set at the nursing unit ready to be used, and two sets in active storage for weekends or emergency use.

The hospital laundry serves a large segment of the hospital. The patient care units need linen. The operating room uses a vast supply of clean linens. The delivery room and imaging department need gowns and drapes. The hospital's central medical supply (central sterile supply), where all of the sterile packs and instruments are wrapped, is a big user of linen. The environmental services department is also a principal customer of the laundry department.

Linen Control and Distribution

A traditional and chronic problem facing hospitals is effective linen control. Without the proper amount of linen at the proper time, patient care, employee morale, and economic hospital operations are all negatively affected.

One of the tasks in dealing with linen control is establishment of regular operating levels, or par levels. A par level is a level of linen inventory required for a specific period in a certain area. In a patient care unit, par levels are usually planned on either a daily or a weekly basis. Linen control is done through controlling par levels on the patient care unit. Another factor in linen control, especially in guarding against pilferage, is that the hospital linen should be properly marked. Linen marking (that is, a hospital name or symbol woven or stamped onto the items) is a very effective means of controlling loss through pilfering. Decals are often affixed to the items. It is common for hospitals to use different-colored linen throughout the hospital. For example, the operating room may use green, maternity may use light blue or pink, and medical-surgical patient care units may use patterned linens.

There are two methods of distributing linen to the nursing units. Clean linen for the day should be on the nursing floor ready to use no later than the start of the first shift (7:00 a.m.). Distribution is handled in a centralized fashion in which one or more large linen carts are regularly rotated around the nursing units from floor to floor. Another method of distributing linen, the decentralized way, is to provide each patient care unit with its own separate linen cart. Through this method, a patient care unit may have a small supply of emergency linens on the floor with the bulk of the linens kept in supervised and/or locked linen carts.

MAINTENANCE DEPARTMENT

A department in the hospital that is often unseen by patients and visitors is maintenance. This is especially true in a new, modern hospital. It is difficult to imagine that there would be much maintenance involved in repairing equipment, buildings, or grounds in a new facility. Yet when one looks at some older hospitals, the role that maintenance has in keeping the hospital operating properly becomes apparent. Hospital equipment and buildings were once relatively simple. With the increased complexity of hospital facilities and equipment, the role of maintenance has become more complex and an additional burden has been placed on the maintenance function of the hospital.

Functions

The traditional or primary function of the maintenance department is to maintain the buildings and machinery of the hospital. This includes the hot water and steam plant, plumbing, waste disposal systems, and the hospital's electrical power system (including the emergency power systems), as well as the repair of hospital furniture and the upkeep of painting and wall coverings of the interior and exterior of the hospital. Additionally, the department may be responsible for the maintenance of the grounds and for proper landscaping, including snow removal.

Preventive maintenance is work done on a regular basis to keep the hospital in sound repair and to keep machinery and equipment from breaking down. It includes prescheduled inspections, maintenance, minor adjustments, and standard repair. Record keeping is critical to an adequate preventive maintenance program; records should include the purchase date of each item, major repairs on equipment, and inspection reports.

A work order is the key document in maintenance control. It functions to plan, estimate, schedule, and control labor. Examples of items on a work order include the date service is requested, the date it is needed, a work order number, the equipment required, materials required, the number of estimated hours, a brief job description, and the name of the supervisor.

Some hospitals utilize computerized preventive maintenance programs as well as automated systems for processing work orders. Computerization enables the maintenance department to respond quickly and more efficiently to complaints and requests.

Contract maintenance is the use of outside maintenance experts to repair hospital equipment. Traditionally, this is done for large, complex pieces of equipment such as elevators. Nevertheless, as hospitals become more complex with esoteric clinical equipment, outside maintenance specialists are increasingly called upon to supplement the regular maintenance staff. Outside experts usually service imaging equipment. The cost of these repairs could rightfully be included in the cost of hospital maintenance, even though they may show up as a direct expense in the clinical department.

Hospital renovations may also be done through the maintenance department. With the high costs of new construction, renovations have become common practice for hospitals. However, renovation can be just as expensive as new construction where there is inadequate management planning and staffing. The maintenance department must also be concerned with energy conservation since hospitals are in operation seven days a week and use intense energy utilizing machines—such as sterilizing units in the central sterile supply and CT and MRI units in the imaging department.

PLANT ENGINEERING

The plant engineering department is responsible for operating the hospital's power plant or boiler room section. The department is primarily concerned with production and transmission of heat, cool air, the hospital's medical vacuum system, power, and light.

Many hospitals generate some of the energy necessary for critical functions within the hospital, including generating steam for heating systems, hot water, and sterilizing. In addition, it is common for those hospitals that have laundries to generate their own energy for this function. The engineering department, through its power plants, may be involved in cogeneration of steam and electricity. Standby electrical systems for emergency power are also this department's responsibility. Most power plants have a standardized chiller or air conditioning capabilities.

The hospital boiler room is under the direction of a boiler engineer. Many states and cities have licensure laws that require boiler engineers to undergo examinations by a board or a qualified group. In these cases, after passing qualification examinations, the boiler engineer receives an operating license. This license must be posted in the hospital's power plant as proof of the individual's qualifications. The engineering license primarily covers boiler operations, refrigeration, and the fundamentals of other activities related to the power plant.

PARKING FACILITIES

All hospitals need parking facilities. It may fall to the maintenance department to operate and maintain parking facilities. Convenient, safe, and adequate parking can be a big marketing plus for any hospital. Adequate parking facilities can also be helpful in recruiting medical staff and employees. For hospitals in high crime areas, a well-lighted, secure parking facility is necessary in order to retain qualified staff. The most acute need for parking usually occurs during the half-hour overlap time before the change of day shift (7:00 a.m. to 3:30 p.m.) and the half-hour overlap time before the evening shift (3:00 p.m. to 11:30 p.m.).

There are generally three types of parking areas: surface parking, or on-ground parking; multilevel parking, or above-ground parking; and subterranean parking or below-ground parking. Surface parking is the least costly while subterranean parking is the most costly. The enormous growth in outpatient activity has put a tremendous strain on hospitals to provide sufficient parking spaces. The provision of adequate parking areas is especially crucial for urban hospitals that tend to be landlocked. As a result, multilevel parking garages have become popular.

SECURITY

In smaller hospitals, security often falls under the responsibility of the maintenance department, while in larger hospitals security has its own department. It was common until the terrorism act of September 11, 2001, for a retired police officer to be in charge of the security department. Now the department is usually manned by sophisticated security contract services. An effective security program is important not only to secure the hospital's building and equipment, but also to protect the welfare of patients (especially newborns), employees, and visitors. Hospitals bear the liability for unsafe security measures.

GENERAL SAFETY

The hospital should have an overall safety plan, headed by a safety and occupational health director. In smaller hospitals, this is an extra duty of the maintenance director or human resources director.

The safety plan should contain a written safety policy signed by the hospital administrator and should be clearly communicated to all employees. This plan should designate a safety committee comprised of employees and physicians; this committee should meet often. Each hospital department should also have its own safety policies.

It is the duty of the safety director and department director to conduct frequent training and to review accidents and incidents of employees, patients, and visitors in order to prevent similar happenings.

Common employee accidents, nearly all preventable, include needle sticks, back injuries, slips and falls, and electrical shocks. Common injuries to patients include falls from beds and same-surface falls. Visitor slips and falls also occur.

The Occupational Safety and Health Administration (OSHA) is the governmental body established in 1970 charged with safeguarding the health and safety of all employees. Enforcement of standards, exposure limits for hazardous materials, accident reporting, and safety training are aspects of OSHA. Its Web site is available at http://www.OSHA.gov.

Safety can also be a medical issue. Special committees such as the pharmacy and therapeutic committee should track safety issues such as incorrect medication dosages or medication given to the incorrect patient.

Should an injury occur to an employee, patient, or visitor, one should summon immediate help, make apologies, and file a written report with the safety director. Training should prevent future occurrences; reports will help to identify patterns, which indicates where additional training is needed.

Safety Programs in Hospitals

A safety program in a hospital is an important part of any hospital, or for that matter, any organization. It can preserve lives, prevent injury, and in the end, save money for the hospital—and it is the right thing to do.

A safety program should contain many things, but the bedrock for all hospital programs is top management support. Without this support, the program will have no seriousness or effectiveness.

Important Elements

Each hospital should have a written safety policy from top management—a policy might read:

> Nothing is as important as the safety of our patients, visitors, and employees. We value everyone's life and cannot waste valuable human resources by allowing injuries, lost time accidents, or repairing equipment damaged through accident or misuse—we must all insure that jobs will be done correctly the first time, with care, and with each employee following safe and healthful procedures. It is paramount that employees safeguard our patients, visitors, and each other through the use of correct procedures and the use of proper safety equipment, and that each employee thinks before acting.

A basic element of a safety program is regular safety meetings conducted within each department. Each hospital department is different; hazards in dietary are not the same hazards found in nursing, and therefore it is important that each department be aware of its uniqueness and takes steps to safeguard its employees through awareness. For example, in nursing, many nurses are injured by needle sticks and many nurses encounter back injuries from incorrectly lifting patients. A good safety program can build awareness of these issues and reduce them through proper training.

Large numbers of injuries occur in the patient population, primarily through falls from beds. Simply instructing the nursing staff always to erect patient bed rails can prevent this. Another problem to patients is medication errors. The nursing staff must be instructed to give the right dose to the right patient at the right time. Checking wristbands is such a simple thing that can save lives.

The safety director should build safety awareness among employees and should investigate each accident when it occurs. The results of a proper investigation can be entered in the hospital loss-prevention system to help prevent future accidents of the same nature. It is important not to punish an employee who has an accident but to learn from the circumstance and to prevent a recurrence.

Safety equipment may be found in the engineering and maintenance department—it may be goggles, a hard hat, or steel toed shoes—and usually it isn't popular with the rank and file employee. Complaints can range from "it's hot" and "it isn't convenient," to "it isn't cool-looking." Management must stress that safety equipment can reduce injury, is required by OSHA, and is in the employee's best interest.

In other areas of the hospital, safety equipment stretches further to include disposable gloves, containers for used-needles and other sharp instruments, and face shields to be worn during surgery by all of the OR team. Today it is impossible to tell by a glance which patient may have HIV, Hepatitis A, B, or C. All patient-contact employees should take "universal" precautions, a term meaning to act as though every patient has a communicable disease.

Top management's support, demonstrated by a written safety policy, regular safety meetings coupled with correct training, the use of safety equipment, and correct accident investigation form the basis of stopping accidents, preventing losses, and keeping patients, visitors, and employees safe and accident free.

FIRE SAFETY

Besides the security department or maintenance department being responsible for fire safety, each work unit must be trained in preventing fires, fighting fires, and evacuating patients. Because most patients are unable to evacuate rapidly from a hospital, hospital facilities have smoke detectors, alarm systems, sprinkler systems, and doors that close automatically to contain the spread of fire, smoke, heat, and gases. Hospitals need to understand current regulations pertaining to fire safety and must implement periodic staff training and fire drills.

DISASTER PLANNING

Hospitals have the duty to save lives—it is essential that they undertake disaster planning for the inevitable day when a disaster occurs. It is also essential that hospitals know that planning alone does not go far enough; the hospital must conduct periodic drills to practice the plan.

Hurricane Katrina, which caused extreme damage to parts of Louisiana, Mississippi, and Alabama in September 2005, proved this point. Countless studies and articles pointed to the fact that New Orleans would not be able to withstand a category 4 or 5 hurricane, yet preparedness seemed to be a secondary thought. In the July 18, 2005, issue of *U.S. News and World Report*, Dan Gilgoff reported about a study conducted by Ivor van Heerden, director of Louisiana State University's Center for the Study of Public Health Impacts of Hurricanes, saying, "if a hurricane comes next month, New Orleans could no longer exist." This proved nearly true, yet many healthcare organizations and hospitals had done little to prepare.

Was everyone unprepared? One group that set an example was the professionals that planned for a "surge" hospital to be assembled quickly in the Pete Marivich Center at Louisiana State University. These professionals prepared by simulating and practicing beforehand with hypothetical "Hurricane Pam," drilling for an event that they believed was likely to occur one day. When the real Hurricane Katrina did blow in, this group erected an 800-bed hospital in the athletic center within hours and accepted casualties immediately, in fact they had to persuade FEMA authorities to send them victims; few in FEMA believed anyone could possibly be ready so quickly. Planning made the difference.

The Joint Commission on Accreditation of Healthcare Organizations and diverse state hospital licensing agencies mandate that hospitals have a written emergency preparedness program to manage natural disasters or emergencies that disrupt the ability to provide care and treatment. The program should include a description of the hospital's role in community-wide preparedness and the hospital's plan to implement specific procedures. It should have provisions for managing space, supplies, communications, and security; it should delineate staff responsibilities and functions; and it should have provisions for managing patients, staff emergency training, and semiannual practice drills.

Types of Internal and External Disasters

Disasters can be categorized in two general ways; internal disasters and external disasters. Internal disasters have various forms, and external disasters have two categories—major and minor.

One form of an internal disaster may occur in the form of a small fire or a collapsed wall due to an earthquake. Employees and outside professionals will respond to the disaster; usually patients are not evacuated unless in immediate danger.

A second form of internal disaster is one in which a *portion* of the hospital's patients, visitors, or employees must be evacuated—this could be a larger fire or some process that renders a section of the hospital unsafe or unusable. The remainder of the hospital continues to function.

A third form is the loss or potential loss of the hospital, and every individual is evacuated. This may be from an impending hurricane, a tornado that has devastated major portions of the hospital, or a flood that has collapsed the emergency power supply of the hospital. An example of this was a recent flood in Houston, Texas. The flood knocked out the city's power supply and the affected hospital had emergency generators located in its underground area, which also promptly flooded, knocking out all power to the hospital. Employees using flashlights evacuated patients, strapped to gurneys, down stairwells. Compounding the problem, some patients were on ventilators and had to be manually resuscitated during the process. The hospital now has taken steps to improve its emergency power system.

A minor external disaster occurs when the hospital receives perhaps 6 to 10 patients—a reasonable number—but the emergency department becomes strained, and physicians then are summoned to report to the hospital. The duration of the crisis is short.

A major external disaster occurs when a hospital is overwhelmed and can no longer safely take patients; many will have to be diverted to other facilities. A major disaster similar to the Oklahoma City federal building bombing or an airplane crash are examples; in these events, patients could number in the hundreds.

Each type of disaster will have its own type of response. These responses must be practiced repeatedly. Periodically, management should activate the telephone recall system, whether activating beepers or having department employees call each other. In addition, there should be periodic community-wide drills that test the coordinated activity between other community resources (police, fire, National Guard, etc.)—this can literally mean the difference, in the future, between who lives and who dies.

BIOMEDICAL ENGINEERING

Biomedical engineering, also referred to as clinical engineering, involves functions related to medical equipment. Medical equipment, also called clinical equipment, covers the following areas: equipment used for patient diagnosis, such as equipment that measures physiological parameters; clinical laboratory equipment; therapeutic treatment equipment; devices that apply radiant energy to the body; equipment for resuscitation, prosthesis, physical therapy, and surgical support; and patient monitoring equipment.

Functions

The biomedical engineers are responsible for certain tasks, which can be categorized by levels. Level I tasks entail the repair of equipment and related documentation of repair history and repair costs. Level II tasks deal with preventive maintenance. These include electric safety checks, new equipment checks, and equipment preuse preparation. Level III tasks involve management and design and specifically deal with planning, purchasing, installation, design, hazard notification, and safety committee support.

Equipment Maintenance

A hospital must have adequate maintenance for all biomedical equipment because the functioning of this equipment has a direct bearing on patient care and safety. The hospital can take four approaches to maintaining biomedical technical equipment. These may be 1) establishing the hospital's own in-house program, 2) subscribing to and relying on a single commercial vendor to provide services, 3) participating in a shared service arrangement with other hospitals, or 4) using a combination of vendors, manufacturers, representatives, and dealers to provide the maintenance of the equipment. The fourth approach is the most exact, but also the most expensive approach.

Staff

Support personnel who are responsible for working on biomedical equipment are referred to as biomedical equipment specialists. There are two recognized levels of specialists: the first level is that of operation specialist who has little formal training but perhaps a great deal of on-the-job training in the hospital. This specialist sets up, checks, and operates the biomedical equipment. The second level involves a more technically oriented specialist with specific biomedical equipment training. This individual is trained to construct and repair the esoteric equipment. The Association for the Advancement of Medical Instrumentation (AAMI) represents and certifies clinical engineers and biomedical equipment specialists.

CONTRACT MANAGEMENT

All facilities support services tend to lend themselves to contract management. Whether a hospital decides to use a total contract service or in-house staff depends on the following factors: quality of service, availability of in-house personnel, knowledge and skills accessibility, availability of in-house equipment, licensing requirements, cost effectiveness, legal issues, and need to expand services. Contract services may include housekeeping, dietary, pharmacy or even physical therapy. The hospital may contract for a complete turn-key operation with the vendor bringing in their own cleaning equipment or cooking equipment, or they may simply provide a contract supervisor that trains employees in better techniques and work methods. Often a rural hospital may have trouble recruiting a pharmacist, a dietician, or a physical therapist, this is a good but sometimes costly solution.

CHAPTER REVIEW

1. What are sanitary specialists?
2. Why is cleaning a hospital a challenging task?
3. What is hazardous waste and what hazardous waste would you expect to find in a hospital?
4. What are par levels?
5. What are some functions of the maintenance department?
6. What are three types of parking areas?
7. Why is fire safety so important to a hospital? What are some precautions a hospital facility takes to detect and contain fires?
8. What are the elements of a general safety program?
9. What are two ways to categorize disasters?
10. What does a biomedical engineer do?

Chapter 15

Administrative Support Services

Key Terms

ABC analysis	Human Resources
Beeper system	Inventory turnover
Centralized purchasing	Job description
Centralized requisitions	Orientation program
Civil Rights Act	Personnel
Economic order quantity (EOQ)	Position control
Equal Employment Opportunity Act	Public Law 93-360
Full-time equivalents (FTEs)	Purchasing agent
Group purchasing	Taft Hartley Act
Hospital auxiliary	Turnover rate

INTRODUCTION

Patient support services and facilities support services were discussed in Chapters 13 and 14. The third type of support services is administrative support. This chapter will examine the department of materials management, human resources, the volunteer auxiliary, and telecommunications management.

MATERIALS MANAGEMENT DEPARTMENT

Materials management is the management and control of goods and supplies, services and equipment from acquisition to disposition. It involves centralization of procurement, processing, inventory control, receiving, and distribution.

Effective materials management results in the purchase of goods, services, and equipment at the lowest costs and ensures that inventories are monitored and controlled.

Purchasing Section

The hospital purchasing section or department is usually under the direction of a purchasing agent or a materials manager. The purchasing agent has to determine what, when, and how much to purchase for hospital inventories. The purchasing agent seeks out sources of supplies and proper vendors. One key objective of the purchasing section is to acquire quality products at the lowest price possible. The purchasing agent must negotiate or evaluate bids to achieve this objective.

To obtain suitable bids, specifications for each product must be set down, preferably in writing. One of the side benefits a hospital realizes from competitive bidding is that the purchasing agent and department heads requesting an item have to give more thought to the item, its usage, and the standards they require for the item. One of the problems with using only price as a determinant is in the issue of service and of the cost of service contracts. If the product needs repair, whether it be a major piece of equipment or smaller, disposable item, the purchasing agent must demand that the sales and service representatives for that vendor arrive quickly to repair the equipment or come in to discuss the product and its characteristics with the users. Service is a factor that must be weighed along with price in competitive bidding. Competitive bids surely can be successful economic tools for the purchasing department and the hospital.

Centralized Purchasing

There is a belief that centralized control and centralized purchasing builds efficient operations and cost containment in hospitals. Centralized purchasing is done for the entire hospital by a single purchasing department, and it is done to assist each department. It can result in savings through consolidation of departmental needs and by reduction of the number of employees involved in purchasing. Further, central purchasing provides the means for strengthening the purchasing department and for establishing clear purchasing policy.

Shared Purchasing

The concept of shared purchasing power or group purchasing is not new to hospitals. Over the years, there have been experiments and cooperative arrangements. The purpose of these co-op arrangements is to reduce the cost of purchases to hospitals. Group purchasing can be as simple as two hospitals deciding to combine certain purchasing activities in order to obtain lower prices for goods and/or services. However, each hospital should review anticompetitive regulations prior to engaging in this cost savings measure. The issue should be referred to the hospital's attorney to examine the issue of group purchasing arrangements.

Leasing

For the purchase of capital equipment, hospitals have frequently leased equipment rather than purchased it. Leasing allows administrators to obtain equipment without having the needed cash on hand. There are two types of leases: financial and operating. The financial lease usually dictates that the term is no longer than about 80 percent of the expected useful life of the asset. The other type of lease is an operating arrangement whereby the lessee may cancel the contract with due notice. Highly technical medical equipment that may be subject to a high degree of obsolescence is usually acquired in this manner.

Receiving Section

The receiving section ensures that the correct number and type of supplies and equipment are properly received. The section is responsible for checking the condition of the items and notifying the accounting department of the receipt of goods. The accounting department is responsible for scheduling payment to vendors. Supervising these receiving functions generally falls to the purchasing agent or personnel in the purchasing section.

Inventories and Inventory Management

Savings result when inventory levels are reduced so that both money and space can be used for other purchases. The objective is to reduce the inventory level as low as possible without running out of items. Table 15-1 highlights some management tools available for effective inventory control.

Storage and Warehousing

The majority of the hospital's inventory is kept in the main hospital warehouse. Items may be distributed via centralized requisitions, par-level systems, or exchange carts. Using requisitions is a traditional system whereby individual departments or patient care units determine when and how much to order. In the par-level system, personnel from the central supply section department go to each appropriate hospital department and patient care unit, count supplies, write up orders, obtain supplies, and bring them back to the unit. Supplies are brought up to standard or par level. A variation of the par-level system is to distribute supplies on a movable cart. According to a predesignated schedule, depleted carts are exchanged with full carts. This is called an exchange cart system.

Table 15-1 Typical Inventory Management Tools

Tool	Formula	Description	Purpose
Inventory turnover	$$\frac{\text{Annual dollar value of items}}{\text{Average inventory value}}$$	Determine how fast items are moving, on average inventory turnover should be 12×/year.	Identify obsolete, slow-moving, or excess items.
Economic order quantity (EOQ)	The square root of the equation $$\frac{(\text{Annual usage} \times 2 \times \text{order cost})}{(\text{annual carrying cost of the unit})}$$	Determine optimal order quantities for items. annual usage of each item in dollars; determine dollar costs of placing purchase orders, holding or carrying costs, and average inventory on hand.	Make economic goals and efficient par levels for each inventory item.
ABC analysis		Classify entire inventory into three categories based on yearly dollar usage of items (A=high dollar usage, B=middle dollar usage, C=low dollar usage).	Determine percentage of costs spent on percentage of inventory.

HUMAN RESOURCES DEPARTMENT

Nearly every hospital has an organized human resources department, previously referred to as the personnel department. This is a very important department when one considers that more than 50 percent of the cost of operating a hospital is usually in labor. This department oversees the maintenance of personnel records and benefits, and it often guides and consults top management of the hospital. This is particularly true now in the age of increased employee record keeping responsibilities and legal requirements placed upon hospitals by federal and state governments and other regulatory agencies.

Department Functions

The human resources department coordinates the processes of selecting and hiring personnel and assists departments in their recruiting and selection needs. The department's activities generally are divided into at least four functional areas: attracting, interviewing and hiring employees, maintaining employees' records and programs once they are within the hospital organization, and insuring that the hospital comply with applicable legal regulations. These functions can include:

- Maintaining a position control plan
- Job analysis
- Creating job descriptions
- Recruitment
- Arranging interviews
- Conducting orientation programs
- Motivation and job enrichment
- Dealing with troubled employees

Maintaining a Position Control Plan

The position control plan is a management tool that allows the hospital to control the number of full-time equivalent employees (FTEs) on the payroll compared to what was budgeted. A full-time equivalent is the number of hours that a full-time employee would work in a given year—2,080 hours per year, which includes paid vacations or other paid time off. It is the human resources department's responsibility to maintain the master employee file and the employee-position control files.

Job Analysis

Before an employee is recruited, selected, interviewed and hired by the hospital, the human resources department should observe and study the tasks and functions to be performed by the employee, the conditions under which the employee will be working, the training and skills aptitude necessary for the employee, and the requisite abilities to perform the job.

Creating Job Descriptions

Following the job analysis, a job description is written. Job description specifications vary among hospitals. Generally, they include job title, the work department to which the employee will be assigned, an outline of the tasks and duties to be performed, any equipment or special tools to be used, and the individual supervising the position.

Recruitment

Usually advertisements to fill job opportunities are placed in newspapers or trade journals or magazines where they are most likely to attract qualified candidates. Past applications are also reviewed. Advanced techniques for hiring include posting vacancies on the hospital's Web site and reviewing applications received through the site. Potential employees are subsequently invited for an interview.

Arranging Interviews

After human resources employees have interviewed and selected the best applicants, interviews are arranged with the appropriate department head or supervisor. After interviews have been conducted, a candidate is selected and an offer is made. The human resources department should not ordinarily make the final selection; it should act only in an advisory capacity to the department director who is experiencing the vacancy.

Conducting Orientation Programs

Orientation has two basic purposes. Firstly, it allows the new employee to get background information about the hospital and its functions and to see how the employee's job fits and contributes to the hospital's overall mission. The orientation should begin to make the employee feel a real part of the hospital family. Hospitals use different techniques for orienting employees—but most include a general orientation lecture and a general tour of the hospital. Benefits, including life insurance, dental insurance, health care insurance, etc. are explained, and written information is distributed. Policies are explained, and parking stickers and a hospital handbook are issued. Sometimes hospitals assign a temporary buddy to each new employee.

Motivation and Job Enrichment

Once the employee is hired, the task of retaining, motivating, and making the employee feel a part of the hospital begins.

One of the measures that hospitals use to evaluate employee morale and retention is turnover. The turnover rate is calculated by dividing the number of employees who voluntarily separated or were fired in a given month by the number of authorized full-time equivalent employees (FTEs) in the hospital. Turnover rates should be calculated every month, and management should review a graph depicting trends by department.

Dealing with Troubled Employees

Another responsibility of the human resources department is to work with troubled and problematic employees. Those with substance abuse problems should receive referrals to appropriate treatment centers. This is handled through the employee assistance program (EAP). The department also handles grievances concerning employee-employer relations. The human resources department also conducts disciplinary workshops so that rank and file department directors present a unified approach to warnings, write-ups, and discharges; and so that the hospital complies with employment and labor laws.

Salaries, Wages, and Benefits

The human resources department has the job of developing, maintaining, and monitoring a wage and salary program. The establishment of a wage and salary program regularly includes four main steps:

1. Analyze each position, determine skills and education required for the position
2. Place each position in a group classification based on its relative importance to the hospital
3. Assign a salary range to each classification
4. Rate employees according to a designated system

Often area-wide wage and salary surveys conducted by hospital counsels are reviewed.

Hospitals traditionally have offered benefits in addition to a salary in order to recruit and retain personnel. Some of the common fringe benefits that may be paid totally or partially by institutions include life insurance, group hospitalization, pension plans, parking, paid vacations, educational assistance, etc. Some hospitals offer a cafeteria plan for benefits, which allows employees to select their own fringe benefits.

Employee Performance Appraisal

The human resources department guides and supports department directors in rating employees. The rating method may involve a formal rating procedure based upon a supervisor completing a form or writing a report. Employee performance appraisals should reflect an employee's knowledge, skills, behavior, attitudes, and overall contribution. Employee-performance appraisal systems are very specific to each institution.

Hospitals and Unions

In 1936, the AFL-CIO initiated a campaign to organize hospital laborers. The goal was to organize a significant portion of nonprofessional health care workers, including dietary, maintenance, and housekeeping personnel. In 1947, the Taft-Hartley, or Labor-Management Relations Act, was passed. This law denied employees of nonprofit hospitals the right to organize. Congress passed Public Law 93-360 on July 26, 1974, which removed the nonprofit hospital's exception from the Taft-Hartley Act. The National Labor Relations Board (NLRB) categorized four labor units within hospitals: 1) registered nurses; 2) all other professionals, including interns, residents, and medical staff physicians; 3) service and maintenance employees, including business office employees; and 4) the technical workforce, including licensed practical nurses. Not surprisingly, hospital management has been opposed to the concept of labor organization within the hospital. Until 1991, the key battleground had involved the size and nature of bargaining units. The dispute ended in April of that year when the United States Supreme Court upheld the National Labor Relations Board's guidelines allowing up to eight bargaining units for hospital workers.

Occupational Licensure

The ever-increasing application of new medical and scientific technology requires skilled and usually licensed personnel. It is the function of the human resources department to keep abreast of all employees' licenses, such as RNs, LVNs, OTs, PTs, RTs, etc.

THE VOLUNTEER ORGANIZATION

The role of the volunteer organization or auxiliary is to supplement services provided by hospital employees. These invaluable volunteers are found operating switchboards, aiding patients' families and friends at the reception desk, delivering books and magazines to patients, and at times, serving as patient representatives. They may provide nursery service on a day-care basis. They aid the social services department in consoling family members of the terminally ill, and they may perform puppet shows for children in the pediatric unit. Volunteers might function as transportation aides in the imaging or physical therapy departments. Many of them assist hospital management by offering skilled typing services and clerical skills. Another invaluable service operated by volunteers is the gift and flower shop found in many hospitals. Volunteers also represent the hospital at community health fairs by staffing booths where they hand out brochures and assist doctors and nurses who perform free public health tests such as blood pressure, cholesterol, and diabetes screening.

The director of volunteers' responsibilities includes recruiting, interviewing, and arranging volunteer assignments with various functional department heads in the hospital, providing their orientation, and assisting in training. The director is also responsible for maintaining a strong liaison with the department heads with whom the volunteers work and relate. It is the director's job to keep the volunteers informed of pertinent hospital policies and procedures and benefits such as parking and meals. One key issue in volunteer service is the volunteers' authority in the hospital. The authority of volunteers is noted in the hospital's bylaws. In those cases, the bylaws would delineate the functions and purposes of the volunteer effort. The wise administrator or CEO frequently visits during the hospital auxiliary meeting.

TELECOMMUNICATIONS MANAGEMENT

The nerve center for telecommunication functions is the hospital switchboard. Staffed 24 hours a day, this area is a key to public relations for the hospital because it is often the first contact a patient or family member has with the hospital.

Many hospitals have sophisticated, computer-driven beeper systems such as satellite transmission, data communications, and high tech telephone systems. Others still rely on hospital telephone operators to activate the beeper system. Telecommunication systems function to assist the caregivers' availability as well as offering an up-to-date business communications system.

CHAPTER REVIEW

1. What is the function of the materials management department?
2. What does the purchasing agent do?
3. Describe competitive bidding vs. centralized purchasing vs. shared purchasing.
4. Describe a typical position control plan. Why is it important?
5. What is an EAP?
6. What are the two forms of sexual harassment?
7. What does Title VII of the 1964 Civil Rights Act cover?
8. Why are random drug screens and criminal background checks important in preemployment screening?
9. May management require employees to undergo polygraph tests?
10. What are some roles of hospital volunteers?

Part VII
Hospital Finances

Cost Reimbursement

In a cost-reimbursement system, hospitals were paid based on their total costs or reasonable costs. Reasonable costs were determined through an elaborate cost-finding process called the cost report, which was prepared by the hospital at the end of its fiscal year. Many third-party payers, e.g., Medicare, have eliminated this process with methods such as negotiated bids or diagnostic-related groups.

Specific Services/Negotiated Bids

The specific services method of payment was based on charges for specific services, such as laboratory, pharmacy, surgery, and nursing services. Typically, hospital management and the board of directors set the institution's charges. The charges could then be discounted or negotiated. Negotiated bids entail an arrangement between a hospital and a third-party payer. Usually a fee arrangement is set for a specific time, with contracts periodically renegotiated as the hospital incurs increased costs. It was crucial for hospitals to plan and control costs under this type of payment method. Health maintenance organizations (HMOs) and preferred provider organizations (PPOs) used this category.

Diagnostic Related Groups (DRGs)

The prospective payment system, or DRG system of payment, was based on prospectively determined prices or rates rather than retrospectively determined costs. This system evolved from research conducted at Yale University in which related diagnoses were grouped together as predictions for length of stay. This system became universal for Medicare in 1983 following the Tax Equity and Fiscal Responsibility Act of 1982. All patient diagnoses were grouped into hundreds of DRGs with each DRG having a fixed payment. Hospitals were paid on these fixed fees regardless of the costs incurred for treating patients. This caused many facilities to seek ways to get patients out of the hospital quickly through discharge strategies utilizing long-term care facilities, to the patient's own home for scheduled home health visits, or to a hospice for care.

Capitation

Management of the hospital may engage in a capitation arrangement with a third-party payer in order to provide a fixed set of services for a fixed group for a fixed payment per patient. For example, a rural hospital contracts with the

Veterans Administration (VA) and agrees to provide limited health care services to 80 local selected veterans in the following manner:

The 80 veterans receive unlimited consultation with the hospital's physician assistant for 1 year with chest x-rays provided when necessary, at an annual cost of $500 per veteran. The hospital receives a check from the VA for $40,000 at the beginning of the year and bears the risk that the cost of care will not exceed the $40,000. In return, the veterans do not have to drive 200 miles to the nearest VA hospital for simple care. Should a veteran need to be hospitalized or need advanced care such as a CT or MRI, the veteran must drive the 200 miles. However, for simple colds, sprains, etc., he or she can be seen at the local level. If the rural hospital can provide the total yearly care for all 80 in the group at less than $40,000, the hospital makes a profit. However, if the cost of care exceeds the capitated price of $40,000, the hospital has exceeded the risk. The use of these contracts is increasing.

THE MAJOR PAYERS

Medicare

On July 1, 1966, under Public Law 89-97, the Medicare program became effective across the nation. The Medicare program was an outgrowth of federal legislation to meet the growing problems of the aged and the disabled in receiving proper, affordable health services. As part of the Social Security Amendments of 1965 (commonly referred to as Title XVIII), Medicare benefits are to be provided to senior citizens (over the age of 65) under two separate but closely related programs. These programs are referred to as Part A of Title XVIII, which pays for hospital services as well as nursing home care (that is, posthospitalization) and other institutional care, and Part B of Title XVIII (known as supplementary medical insurance), which basically pays for physician fees and certain diagnostic services. The supplementary program, or Part B, is voluntary. After age 65, the beneficiaries can subscribe to this at their own expense.

Since its passage in 1966, Medicare has become generally acceptable to consumers. For the average patient, there are four distinct pluses in the Medicare program:

1. It provides almost universal coverage for the elderly.
2. It usually offers better benefits than any private health insurance program could offer to this age group.
3. It assures senior citizens a certain level of access to quality care institutions.
4. It requires relatively smaller out-of-pocket expenses for the elderly.

Medicaid

Along with Medicare legislation in 1966, Medicaid legislation was enacted under Title XIX of the Social Security Act. The primary purpose of Medicaid legislation was to finance health care services for the poor and medically indigent. However, unlike Medicare, which was universally applied to all citizens over the age of 65, federal law required a qualifying eligibility, *but left it to each of the 50 states* to determine who was disadvantaged or medically indigent and consequently eligible for Medicaid benefits. Each state designs its own health services benefit plan and administers the Medicaid program at the state level. Because Medicaid is a big expense to the states, many have tightened requirements, throwing thousands of former recipients into the unqualified ranks.

Typically, the costs of the Medicaid program are shared by the federal government and the individual states. The big discrepancy in the Medicaid program occurs with outpatient and clinical services (physicians' services). Each state can design its own Medicaid outpatient and physician reimbursement schedules.

Unlike the rather universal popularity of the Medicare program, Medicaid has been beset by critics from all sides since its inception. The principal criticism has focused on the problems of costs and eligibility in the program. As noted, the definition of medical indigence was, at the beginning, left to the individual states. But because certain states, like California and New York, provided rather liberal income limits for participants, the federal government has at times set various upper and lower qualifying limits for various aspects of the program. Accordingly, many have been eliminated from the medically indigent ranks.

Additionally, Medicaid has become in some states a political "football," with back-and-forth debate on increasing or cutting benefits and funding for the program, depending on who wins at the ballot box. Certain states have established a freeze on Medicaid payments until the end of a certain number of years and have set payment ceilings to be determined by the state, in contrast to the nearly open-ended Medicare cost reimbursement formulas.

Blue Cross/Blue Shield

Blue Cross is a nongovernmental, nonprofit corporation that offers an insurance program that covers certain hospital services and pays benefits based on a contract between an individual plan and the Blue Cross insurance program in a particular area. Blue Shield is the same arrangement for the physician component; in other words, it is very similar to the Part B portion of the Medicare legislation. Blue Cross contracts vary substantially in reimbursement; for inpatient care, it is similar to Medicare. Payments to hospitals by Blue Cross represents a major percentage of hospital revenues in some parts of this country.

Blue Cross establishes its premiums based on the average cost of actual or anticipated hospital care used by all of its subscribers within a selected geographic area or a particular industry or company. The rate usually does not vary for different groups or subgroups of Blue Cross subscribers; for example, it does not vary based on claims of experience, age, sex, or health status. This method is referred to as the community rating method. Insurance plans that do not use a community rating method may use an experience-rated plan.

Private Insurance

The fourth major type of reimbursement is used by those patients who employ commercial insurance companies other than Blue Cross to cover their hospitalization. Insurance companies cover hospital services and most contract directly with hospitals for direct payment.

Managed Care Plans

Managed care systems are reimbursement systems that started as a control mechanism for escalating medical care costs. The United States experienced rapid growth in two forms of managed care: health maintenance organizations (HMOs), which provide all services to the enrollee (physicians, laboratory tests, imaging, etc.; and preferred provider organizations (PPOs), which is a listing of physicians who have contractually agreed to treat those that enroll. These programs, utilizing prospective (getting permission before a procedure is done) and retrospective (reviewing each case after the patient is discharged) review efforts, attempt to reduce hospital use and thereby reduce costs. These plans leveled out in popularity around 2002 and are now slightly declining in number. Replacing them today are plans known as consumer-driven plans in which an employee receives a fixed contribution from his/her employer and then purchases the best plan for his or her situation, often paying for a portion of the coverage out of pocket.

Self-Paying Patients

At any one time in the United States, there are approximately 40–45 million people without health insurance. This includes people in job transition who are not yet covered under an employer plan, employees of small companies that do not provide health coverage, people who choose to take the risk of being uninsured, or those who are simply unemployed. Under the federal EMTALA law, if an uninsured patient presents to the ED, hospitals must at least examine him, stabilize him, and, if necessary, transfer him to a more competent facility.

FINANCIAL AND STATISTICAL REPORTS

The budgeting process produces actual and projected financial and statistical statements. Individual hospitals vary on the specific formats of these documents, but generally they include: 1) a revenue and expense statement (or profit and loss) for the period, as shown in see Table 17-1; 2) a balance sheet depicting assets on one side and liabilities and equity on the other side (hence the name balance sheet), as shown in Table 17-2; and 3) a statistical report, as shown in Table 17-3. One common technique used to assess a hospital's financial condition (strength or weakness) is ratio analysis. This involves a focus on key financial relationships of values given within the statement of revenue and expenses (income statement) and the balance sheet. Usually historical comparisons are made, as well as comparisons to industry standards. Table 17-4 explains the four major categories of financial ratios.

Table 17-1 ABC Hospital Statement of Revenue and Expense (Profit and Loss) for June

	Budget	*Actual*	*Variance*
Operating revenue			
Room and board	$540,000	$570,000	$30,000
Professional services	$600,000	$605,000	$5,000
Other operating income	$110,000	$100,000	($10,000)
Gross operating revenue	$1,250,000	$1,275,000	$25,000
Less: Allowances			
Contractual adjustments	$65,000	$70,000	($5,000)
Uncollectible (charity and bad debts)	$20,000	$25,000	($5,000)
Total allowances	$85,000	$95,000	($10,000)
Net operating revenue	$1,165,000	$1,180,000	$15,000
Operating expenses			
Operating costs	$160,000	$180,000	($20,000)
Payroll costs	$550,000	$570,000	($20,000)
Depreciation	$60,000	$60,000	—
Interest	$30,000	$30,000	—
Total operating expense	$800,000	$840,000	($40,000)
Net gain from operations	$365,000	$340,000	($25,000)
Non-operating revenue	$10,000	$10,000	—
Excess of revenue over expenses	**$375,000**	**$350,000**	**($25,000)**

Table 17-2 ABC Hospital Operating Fund: Balance Sheet—June 30, 20XX

Assets		Liabilities	
Category	*Amount*	*Category*	*Amount*
Current assets		Current liabilities	
Cash	$400,000	Notes payable	$200,000
Accounts	$2,500,000	Accounts payable	$350,000
receivable		Accrued expenses	$80,000
Less: Allowance for bad	($100,000)	Third-party advances	$200,000
debts		Accounts payable	$350,000
Contractual Allowances	($300,000)	Current portion long-	$760,000
		term debt	
Net accounts receivable	$2,500,000	Total current liabilities	$1,590,000
Due to/from other funds	$100,000	Long-term debt	
Inventory	$200,000	Mortgage payable	$5,220,000
Prepaid expenses	$30,000	Leases	$810,000
Total other assets	$330,000	Total long term debt	$6,030,0001
TOTAL CURRENT ASSETS	$2,830,000	Total liabilities	$7,620,000
Property, buildings, and			
equipment			
Land	$300,000		
Land improvements	$100,000		
Buildings	$9,000,000		
Fixed equipment	$500,000		
Movable equipment	$300,000		
Less: Accumulated			
depreciation	($2,930,000)		
Net property, building and	$7,270,000	Fund balance	$2,995,000
equipment			
Other assets			
Board-designated assets	$500,000		
Deposits	$15,000		
Total other assets	$515,000	Total liabilities and fund	$10,615,000
Total operating fund assets	$10,615,000	balance	

Statistical Report

The data on a simplified statistical report (Table 17-3) shows the hospital's overall inpatient and key outpatient volumes. Because hospitals have such a high fixed-cost component, management must be sensitive to changes in service volumes. Accordingly, it is important to use this statistical data to analyze operating

Table 17-3 ABC Hospital: Statistical Report for the Two Months Ended August 31, 20XX

	Current month	Prior month
Operating statistics		
Patient days	4,100	4,000
Maximum days per licensed capacity (150 beds)	4,500	4,500
Percentage of occupancy	91	89
Average census	137	134
Average length of stay (for discharges)	7.5	7.3
Admissions	540	545
Emergency department visits	1,200	1,100
Outpatient visits	900	1,000
Per patient day		
Gross operating revenue	$1256.00	$1250.00
Total operating costs	$1213.00	$1210.00

Table 17-4 Financial Ratios

Category	Purpose	Example
Liquidity ratios	Measure the hospital's ability to meet its short-term maturing obligations.	$\text{Current ratio} = \dfrac{\text{Current assets}}{\text{Current liabilities}}$
Capital structure	Assess the hospital's long-term solvency or liquidity and ability to increase debt financing.	$\text{Long-term debt to equity ratio} = \dfrac{\text{Long-term debt}}{\text{Fund balance}}$
Activity ratios	Measure the relationship between the hospital's revenue and assets and indicate efficiency.	$\text{Total asset turnover} = \dfrac{\text{Total operating revenue}}{\text{Total assets}}$
Profitability ratios	Indicate the hospital's level of net income.	$\text{Operating margin ratio} = \dfrac{\text{Net operating ratio}}{\text{Total operating revenue}}$

costs and operating revenue. It is common to display hospital per patient day costs and revenue amounts for a given period.

Capital Formation

There are three primary sources for financing hospital construction and major equipment: 1) equity: using the hospital's own funds from retained profits; 2) debt: the hospital borrows the funds, e.g., through mortgage financing; and 3) the receipt of contributions, including fund raising. With respect to debt financing most hospitals usually have a lead bank from which the hospital may obtain a loan or establish a line of credit. In mortgage financing, the mortgage is placed with a bank or other lending institution. A popular option for hospitals to obtain debt financing is to issue or float a bond. Not-for-profit hospitals are permitted to use tax-exempt revenue bonds (bonds which are tax-free, issued by hospitals to generate capital, usually for long-term building projects). Most hospital bonds are given credit ratings, which assess the bond's relative risk. The two primary bond-rating agencies are Moody's and Standard & Poor's which issue opinions of the credit worthiness of the bonds, usually as "A-rated," "B-rated," etc., an indicator of how likely the institution is to default on repayment.

Capital Budgets

The advanced purchase of equipment such as MRI machines or CT scanners must be well planned. Hospitals prepare special budgets called capital budgets. These reflect the equipment costs and often the service contract costs, and they will project the revenue per procedure and the expected number of procedures, then conclude with the expected payback period. Due to the large capital outlay required, many hospitals often choose to lease rather than purchase such equipment. An added advantage is that at the end of the lease, the hospital either can choose to make a balloon payment and purchase the equipment, or it can relinquish the equipment, instead choosing to lease or purchase advanced technology.

CHAPTER REVIEW

1. What is budgeting? What are three types of budgeting?
2. What are the four steps in building an operating budget?
3. What is a balance sheet?
4. What is the difference between debt and equity financing?
5. What is a capital budget?

6. Why do some hospitals choose to lease rather that purchase large capital equipment?
7. Describe four types of financial ratios and for what reason each is used.
8. What is equity capital? How is it accumulated and for what is it used?
9. Who should be involved in the budgeting process? Why should finance personnel not be the only ones involved?

Chapter 18

Business Functions

Key Terms

Accounts receivable

Accrual accounting

Chart of accounts

Chief financial officer (CFO)

Collection agency

Corporate compliance

Fund accounting

Management information system
  (MIS)

Online management reports

Posting entries

INTRODUCTION

We have looked at two of the three major financial functions of the hospital. In Chapter 16, we identified where and how the hospital receives its revenue. In Chapter 17, we have analyzed how a hospital structures its budgets for operations, cash, and capital equipment. In this chapter, we will review the internal hospital business functions.

The hospital's functions and responsibilities in this area include: 1) the maintenance of adequate accounting systems for all income and expenditures; 2) the development and coordination of the budget control mechanism; 3) credit and collections procedures; 4) collection of cash and banking procedures; 5) the maintenance of internal controls; 6) the compilation of pertinent departmental statistics in conjunction with the medical records department; and 7) the preparation of financial reports that can be invaluable tools for the chief financial officer (CFO). The CFO reports directly to the CEO. A CFO's responsibilities extend to all phases of financial management of the hospital, including general accounting and bookkeeping, patient accounts, and various aspects of financial reporting. Under the CFO, there is a business office manager, and there is possibly a patient accounts manager, as well as a senior accountant (the individual in charge of the accounting division). The CFO consults frequently with the CEO and the numerous hospital department heads. The CFO's knowledge of all phases of the hospital's finances provides a basis for recommending ways to improve the hospital's services. Recently, CFOs have been emphasizing ways to decrease costs and improve third-party reimbursement. These skilled professionals are experts in analyzing data and inspecting reports. Through these accounting records, from which the financial statements are prepared, the hospital can determine its financial soundness.

THE ACCOUNTANT

In order to provide uniformity throughout the industry, hospitals usually follow the uniform classification of accounts shown in the American Hospital Association's "chart of accounts" for hospitals. The hospital accountant is usually the principal person assigned the responsibility for the hospital's accounting system. The accountant must be familiar with the current accounting procedures and statistical financial analyses used in the hospital field. The accountant reports to the CFO and works closely with patient accounts and billing in the financial information system department. The senior accountant supervises the recording (posting) of entries in hospital ledgers and trial balances to ensure accuracy of the records. In addition, these entries are audited annually at random by an external firm. Generally, the accountant completes any tax statements the hospital must submit and files cost reports with insurers.

HOSPITAL ACCOUNTING

Even though the hospital may be a nonprofit institution, it must adhere to strict accounting rules. The accounting records are, in the final analysis, the reports that express in dollars and cents the financial status of the hospital. Not all hospital accounting is uniform. However, with the passage of Medicare legislation in 1966, many hospitals now account for their activities in very similar ways. Indeed, the similarities between hospitals are much more apparent than their individual peculiarities.

Fund Accounting

Hospital accounting is sometimes called fund accounting. This type of accounting was adopted by hospitals because they are the beneficiaries of many philanthropic efforts in the community. Since hospitals may be the recipients of endowment funds and gifts for very special purposes, it is necessary for them to have more than one fund. Establishment of these individual funds places the hospital and its board in a fiduciary position that must adhere to the strict wishes of the donor. In order to carry out this responsibility, it has been necessary to separate endowment funds and gifts from other assets of the hospital.

In fund accounting, each distinct phase of financial activity is handled as a separate accounting entry with its own particular objective. Each of the separate funds, or accounts, is self-balancing. Fund accounting is a technique that accounts for separate entities in a single hospital or institution. Each separate fund represents a distinct phase of the hospital's financial obligations and operations. The hospital is legally responsible for a separate accounting of each of these funds.

Most nonprofit hospitals have four distinct funds, or basic sets of books, that are interrelated. These are the general fund, the plant fund, the endowment fund, and the special fund. For the employee and the community, the operations of the hospital appear to be reflected in the general fund. This fund has several categories, including assets, liabilities, net worth, income, total income expenses (those expenses used to generate income for the hospital), and net gain or loss. Income includes gross income, which comes from reimbursements and allowances, such as contractual adjustments; net income; and other income, which frequently comes from nonoperations, such as gift shops and interest income. A major component of total income expense is salaries and wages, which in many hospitals is about one-half of the total operating expenses, as was discussed earlier. The fund also reflects the net gain or loss for the accounting period. The hospital's operating fund is an account for the hospital's day-to-day financial activities that are not required to be accounted for in any separate or special fund or subcategory group. It is the most active fund in the hospital.

Hospitals generally operate on an accrual basis of accounting. Under this system, income is recorded in the period in which it is earned, as opposed to a cash basis, under which income is recorded when cash is received. Similarly, the accrual basis provides for the recording of expenses in the period in which they are incurred and for the recording of assets in the period in which they are acquired. In a cash basis method, the recording of expenses and asset acquisitions is made at the time the cash is disbursed for each item. It is important to understand these two approaches to accounting. The accrual basis method is more accurate and more complete.

MANAGEMENT INFORMATION SYSTEMS (MIS)

The age of computers in the hospital field began in the mid-1950s, and the use of computers has since increased rapidly to include all hospitals. Though there has been great progress toward the use of a total management information system (MIS) and other applications, the most sophisticated may be in the financial area.

For this reason, hospitals may have a separate financial information department under the guidance of the CFO.

Business statistics either are recorded at the department level or received from each department on a computer disc to be entered directly into the hospital's computer network. From these statistics and patient charges, patients' bills are generated. As a byproduct, hosts of important statistical and online management reports are also developed, which could include revenue percentages generated from insurance, Medicare, or Medicaid. After the patient accounting system has been entered into the computer, the rest of the accounting system of the hospital (starting with the hospital's general ledger) can also be entered. Other financial-related activities include the hospital's payroll and the hospital's purchasing and inventory control system. Networked computers mean greater control over collection activities, reduced patient accounts receivable (the fewer days in accounts receivable the better—hospitals want to collect money owed them quickly), improved cash flow, and improved customer service relations.

The trend in management information systems has been toward networked departments, using optical (paperless) storage. It will eventually be wireless. In addition to financial functions, hospitals are increasingly using information systems in planning decisions with regard to medical records, administrative research, the laboratories, nursing activities, marketing, and patient care activities.

THE PUBLIC ACCOUNTING FIRM

Traditionally, hospitals have hired certified public accounting (CPA) firms to conduct an annual audit of the hospital's financial reports. The auditing firm monitors the hospital's internal controls, verifies the values of the hospital's assets, and traces accounting transactions. The firm gives a second opinion on the hospital's financial situation. It generates its own annual financial reports, which are referred to as the certified statements or audited financials. Firms issue a management letter that accompanies the financial reports. The management letter describes for the board and administration those financial areas that require corrective action. In the era of heavy third-party reimbursement, the auditors can aid hospitals that are seeking to maximize their reimbursements.

PATIENT ACCOUNTS AND BILLING DEPARTMENT

The traditional hospital business office has essentially become the patient accounts and billing department. The primary functions of this department are to manage patient accounts, hospital accounts, and receivables, and to monitor patient bills. Patient account management includes interviewing patients to gather information on credit and collection potential, e.g., employment history, insurance coverage, deductibles, and coinsurance. Insurance claims need to be submitted by the hospital on a timely basis to third-party payers. Many hospitals use automated systems for claim submission. The department is also responsible for maintaining accurate billing records, checking amounts received against patient bills, comparing bills to hospital rates to ensure accuracy, sending out itemized statements to patients, and showing payments received and balances due. Often the hospital cashier's function is part of the patient accounts and billing department.

When delinquent patient accounts cannot be collected, they are often referred to a collection agency for further collection effort. The agency usually attempts to collect bills the hospital has given up on, taking a percentage of the collected amount. Hospitals need to evaluate the cost and benefits of using a collection agency for unpaid patient accounts. Not surprisingly, patients frequently question and/or complain about their bills. A critical role for the patient accounts and billing department is to maintain positive customer relations. The department is responsible for explaining billing procedures and forms, handling patient complaints, and resolving patients' billing problems.

CORPORATE COMPLIANCE PROGRAMS

Due to numerous and complex laws and regulations, most health care organizations have instituted a corporate compliance program. The program is designed to audit and investigate internal programs to ensure that violations of laws and regulations are prevented, whether they are criminal or not. A senior person in the organization is given responsibility for the program and sets up monitoring and auditing systems to ensure compliance and deter criminal conduct. Policies and procedures are written and communicated so that all employees understand the bright line between compliance and noncompliance. If offenses are detected, the compliance officer and organization must respond appropriately to correct the offense and prevent similar offenses.

CHAPTER REVIEW

1. What are five major business functions of a hospital?
2. What is fund accounting?
3. What are some trends in hospital MIS?
4. What is reviewed in an annual audit?
5. What is the function of the patient accounts and billing department?
6. What are the reasons that a hospital may use an outside CPA firm?

7. What are the duties and responsibilities of the corporate compliance officer? To whom should he or she report?

8. A patient demands an itemized bill from your hospital and then complains to you that she was charged $129.00 for a "mucus collection system" which turned out to be a box of tissues. How do you respond to her complaint?

Part VIII
Evaluating Care

Chapter 19

Medical Records

INTRODUCTION (HIPAA)

The hospital medical record has undergone great changes. These changes are due to greater demand and use of the information contained in the medical record. The upsurge of interest in the medical record has been aided by an increase in complexity of medical care and the renewed interest in information carried in the medical record. There are demands from third-party payers and requirements based on federal and state legislation that have increased the need for access to the patient's medical record.

Hospitals are required to conduct utilization reviews and medical audits that use the medical record. The computer, as a tool in the health information and management system, is frequently interfaced with the patient's medical record. This has created a completely new discipline and scientific approach in handling the record. All of these factors have added to the growth and complexity of the hospital's medical records department. Added to this is an increased concern for patient confidentiality and the recent passage of the Health Insurance Portability and Accountability Act of 1996 (HIPAA) to ensure such. The HIPAA, Public Law

104-191, was signed into law by President Bill Clinton on August 21, 1996. It had four primary objectives, which were:

1. To assure health insurance portability by eliminating job-lock due to pre-existing conditions.
2. To reduce health care fraud and abuse.
3. To guarantee security and privacy of health information.
4. To enforce standards for health information.

The third item drew the most attention from hospitals and physicians' offices. There are two important rules—the *security rule* and the *privacy rule*—that work to safeguard *protected health information* (PHI).

PHI is defined as health information that 1) identifies or could identify an individual; 2) is created by an entity that is covered by HIPAA (such as hospitals and physicians' offices and their business partners); 3) is transmitted or maintained in any medium (electronic or otherwise); and 4) relates to past, present, or future care of a person or the payment for the care provided.

The major goal of the privacy rule is to properly protect the individual's health information while still allowing the flow of health information needed to provide high quality health care. Though the security rule only deals with electronic health information, this is a moot point because the privacy rule still requires appropriate security for PHI, no matter the format. Within the security rule are requirements for *physical* safeguards to protect information from disclosure, modification, or destruction. Also included are *technical* safeguards to control access to systems that contain PHI. There is also a chain of trust partner agreement requirement for business associates that could create, receive, maintain, or transmit PHI on behalf of the entity. Documents must be maintained for 6 years.

HIPAA also added strength to the government's effort to fight health care fraud and abuse. The act provided new civil and criminal enforcement tools, and it provides a coordinated framework for local, state, and federal law enforcement agencies. To date, the act has been successful in increasing the investigation and successful prosecution of health care fraud in the United States.

To view more about the act, please see http://www.cms.hhs.gov/hipaa.

PURPOSE OF THE MEDICAL RECORD

The purpose of the medical record is to document the course of the patient's illness and treatment (medical care) during a particular period and during any subsequent period as an inpatient or outpatient. There are manual and electronic medical records.

MANUAL MEDICAL RECORDS

Traditionally, the medical record has been a collection or package of hand-written or typed notes, forms, and/or reports. The forms are the vehicle for the physician and health providers (nurses, physical therapists, respiratory therapists, dieticians, etc.) to record the patient's illness and course of recovery. This includes the patient's admission form, medical history, physical examination, and labora-tory, imaging and special report forms. If the patient undergoes surgery, there is a signed authorization and consent form obtained prior to surgery. The patient's anesthesia record will be attached to the surgeon's operative report, which is dic-tated and typed. Frequently, physicians' orders will follow the admission form. These orders are on forms, maintained in chronological fashion, by which the physician communicates to nurses and other health care professionals the instruc-tions for determining the patient's diagnosis and carrying out needed therapy. Usually near the physician's order sheets are progress note sheets. The progress note sheets are often the largest part of any patient's medical record. The nurses' notes or nursing records are really progress notes from a nursing viewpoint. The nursing notes contain the nurses' around-the-clock observations of the patient. Finally, a discharge order written by the physician indicating that the patient can be discharged is included in the record. Within a day or two of the discharge of a patient, it is required that the physician dictate a narrative summary of the patient's stay. The summary is required for several reasons: 1) patient billing can-not send a bill until the summary is complete; 2) a summary is useful for care-givers if the patient must be quickly readmitted; and 3) the Joint Commission places great importance on this in their survey because it is an indicator of patient care. The summary is typed and placed into the medical record after the patient has left the hospital. Although this is the last document recorded by the physician, it is generally placed in first position when the record is finally stored so that reviewers can quickly see the course of the patient's hospital stay. All these forms and reports are contained in a one-unit record (single) folder called a chart.

ELECTRONIC MEDICAL RECORDS

Today more and more hospitals are replacing manual medical records with electronic medical records, which are optical disk devices resembling CDs. Paper medical records are scanned onto these disks to foster faster retrieval, fewer errors, and of course, much less storage space. Automation has made it possible to capture, store, retrieve, and present clinical data. Many computers offer online systems that provide hospital staff with direct access to computerized databases through decentralized communication terminals. Some hospitals have personal computers (PCs) at the patients' bedsides, while others have PCs at the nurses' workstations. Ideally, the computerized system for medical records should be integrated with the hospital's information system.

One of the benefits of electronic medical records is that the records are organized and legible and, therefore, likely to minimize misunderstandings or patient case errors. The major advantage of computerization, however, is multiple accesses by various users simultaneously; these users do not have to wait for a transcribed, printed copy. Health care professionals, especially nurses, are more productive when less time is devoted to paperwork. Computerization can enhance the operations of the medical records department. This is especially true of functions like coding, abstracting, noting chart deficiencies, and correspondence.

Automation also helps expedite the process of completing medical records, which will improve the timely submission of patient bills. In addition, by computerizing selected clinical data in the patient record, the hospital will be able to track and detail clinical information quickly and efficiently. One of the most important aspects to be considered when developing and implementing a computerized system is getting user acceptance early. The acceptance process should begin with the planning stage. User acceptance increases the level of comfort that health care professionals feel while using a sophisticated computerized system. The information system must also be secure. Restricted access prevents unauthorized use; correct software and hardware make alterations impossible. Changes are always added, but alterations, strikeovers, or deletions are *never* allowed.

THE MEDICAL RECORDS DEPARTMENT

Medical records have been retained for hundreds of years, even before pencil and paper were invented. We can assume that some of the hieroglyphics on Egyptian tombs and temples referred to medical aspects of the deceased. A new impetus in medical records departments and medical records administration was launched early in the 1900s. In 1912, medical records librarians gathered at Massachusetts General Hospital to discuss their common interests. In 1928 the Association of Record Librarians of North America was born. This later became known as the American Association of Medical Records Librarians.

The individual in charge of the medical records department is either a registered records administrator or an accredited records technician who has passed the American Medical Association's exam. The department director is called the medical records administrator. Part of the medical records administrator's job is to organize and manage the medical records system and to provide efficient medical records services to the hospital. Specifically, this person's duties include: 1) planning, designing, and technically evaluating patient information; 2) planning, directing, and controlling the administration of the medical records department and its services; 3) aiding the medical staff in its medical records work; 4) developing statistical reports for management and the medical staff; and 5) analyzing technical evaluations of health records and indices.

Hospital medical records are highly visible instruments used in the evaluation of patient care. This being the case, it is common for third parties, and especially the JCAHO, during their annual or triennial surveys, to study and review carefully the patients' medical records.

Though the medical record presents a wealth of data for countless third parties, quality improvement reviewers, and third-party payers, one of the most common problems is that of delinquent medical records. Not all physicians complete their medical records in a timely and accurate manner according to the medical staff bylaws. This tends to be a chronic problem faced by medical records administrators across the country. In the final analysis, the most effective measure against these delinquencies is the temporary suspension of privileges until the physicians complete their records. This is usually done by the chief executive officer or designee, with ratification by the board. In fact, if delinquent record problems are serious, they could jeopardize the hospital's accreditation by the JCAHO.

ORGANIZATION OF THE DEPARTMENT

The organization and staffing of the medical records department reflect in a very straightforward way the tasks and functions of the department. The department is staffed to handle 1) release of information, 2) admission and discharge analyses, 3) medical transcriptions, 4) coding and abstracting (generally this involves diagnostic and procedural coding), 5) storage and retrieval, and 6) gathering statistics for use by the hospital.

Coding and abstracting involve assigning a number to the reason for which the patient has entered the hospital. Third party payers such as Medicare pay based on the code number the patient is assigned. For example, the code 273 might be congestive heart failure, code 112 might be tuberculosis, etc. This is accomplished by a skilled medical records technician summarizing the chart and then assigning a uniform "Diagnostic Related Group" code number for the reason the patient has been admitted.

In the area of statistics and record keeping, the statistical section of the medical records department provides the input to many of the computerized data services that hospitals use to generate computerized patient data profiles. The primary source of this data is the patient's discharge abstract that is submitted to third-party agencies. This data is summarized and stored online. Hospitals can retrieve information when needed. Older hard copy medical records may be stored off site and reclaimed when necessary. Often, state laws mandate a recommended retention period of 3, 10, or 30 years or even permanently in some states, depending on the type of record or document.

The transcription section of the medical records department is an area in which medical transcriptionists type summaries and reports dictated by physicians for filing in the medical record. At one time, many hospitals employed medical transcribers; today, the use of outside transcription services can be the standard. With these outside services, transcription is dictated over the telephone, entered into a computer program, and electronically sent back to the hospital. This system offers the hospital the advantage of not having to deal with and manage various hospital employees. The hospital pays exactly for what it receives in transcription and the outside service relieves the hospital from the task of maintaining a bank of technical transcription equipment and employing qualified transcriptionists. A new trend in larger hospitals is to use international services. For example, the transcription can be sent electronically to India late in the day, and the time difference allows the completed transcription to be ready in the United States the next morning.

THE MEDICAL RECORDS COMMITTEE

The hospital's medical records committee is the liaison between the medical records department and the physicians in the hospital. This committee is charged with the responsibility of reviewing and evaluating the medical records function. These tasks should be performed not less than quarterly. Generally, based on random sampling and recommendations from a variety of medical sources, the committee will review certain records on a regular basis for appropriateness. However, the principal responsibility for quality of peer review rests with the medical staff's audit, utilization, review, and quality improvement committees.

The medical records committee's principal responsibility is to supervise the organization of the record. The committee must review and approve all new medical record forms. In view of the fact that the traditional record is a potpourri of medical forms, this can be a time-consuming task. The committee should evaluate the accuracy of certain record notations relating to management and administrative subjects. For example, if physicians are not writing the discharge diagnosis on the medical record at the proper time or in the proper place, the medical records committee should take corrective action. It is the committee's responsibility to monitor the traditional and chronic problem of physicians' delinquency in completing medical records.

The medical records committee does not generally get involved in making recommendations on management issues in the medical records department. For example filing procedures, medical records coding, storage, microfilming, and preservation of certain sections of the record are responsibilities of the medical records administrator in conjunction with the hospital's management.

LEGAL REQUIREMENTS

The medical records administrator is the custodian of medical records and must be alert to certain legal requirements with regard to the handling and release of medical information and medical records. The maintenance of medical records is governed by the several state and federal acts such as HIPAA (discussed previously in this chapter). Records are retained as part of day-to-day business of the hospital.

Rules for releasing medical information vary from state to state. The medical records administrator must understand the specific statute in the state in which the hospital is located. The medical records administrator is also expected to handle privileged communications with individuals through the courts or various governmental agencies under established hospital policy and to follow state and federal statutes and laws. The medical records administrator is the special guardian of medical records that are in litigation (for example, malpractice suits). In that capacity, the medical records administrator has to testify (orally or in writing) at legal hearings and sometimes in court that the hospital medical record is the accurate document it is purported to be.

MEDICAL RECORDS AND QUALITY IMPROVEMENT

The primary function of medical records is to serve as a communications medium for health care workers and physicians. Another major purpose for medical records is to provide the principal database for performing quality improvement. This key role has made hospital medical records increasingly vital documents.

CHAPTER REVIEW

1. Why has the medical records department become increasingly important?
2. What is HIPAA? What are the four main reasons for its passage and which reason has had the most impact on hospitals?
3. Why must physicians complete their medical records in a timely fashion?
4. How is the medical records department organized?
5. What is the function of the medical records committee?
6. If a documentation (entry) mistake is found in a medical record, can it be changed or altered?

7. Are x-rays and other imaging or laboratory tests part of the medical record? If they are, where are they stored?

DISCUSSION QUESTIONS

1. Research who owns the medical records in your state, and discuss the pros and cons of this arrangement.
2. Research how long a medical record must be kept by a hospital in your state. Discuss whether this is an appropriate time period.

Chapter 20

Quality Improvement

DEFINITION

The "quality" part of quality improvement (originally called "quality assurance") is an often-debated topic in health care. The term "quality" is not all embracing; it may diverge based on who is defining it, and it may vary in hospitals and among physicians. It is usually a *relative term*—in relation to something else.

A traditional view from physicians is that the quality of health care must depend upon the credentials of the provider. There is a belief that the physicians who are highly trained (e.g., cardiologists exploring cardiac problems) are probably better than those who are less well trained (e.g., general practitioners examining cardiac problems). Health care providers also define quality with respect to the technical aspect of care, including the diagnostic and therapeutic aspects of care.

Patients have different views of quality. Patients equate quality with relief of symptoms or with the magazines and furniture in the waiting area—this is because patients do not practice medicine. Quality judging is better left to professional peer groups.

Hospital quality improvement is actually a continuing process. Its goals are to measure and evaluate professional services rendered to the hospital patient. Service in a proper quality improvement program is measured against a prevailing and accepted standard of professional care (remember it was stated that it is a relevant term). The product of quality improvement is the improvement of care; it is intended to change the behavior of physicians and health team members where necessary.

HISTORICAL REVIEW

Quality improvement programs in the United States became common and were better understood following the early 1900s when Abraham Flexner presented his classic report on the quality of medical education in this country. In 1918, the American College of Surgeons initiated the Hospital Standardization Program to encourage uniform medical record formats and to facilitate accurate recording of the patient's medical course. In 1951, based on this effort, the Joint Commission on the Accreditation of Hospitals (JCAH), forerunner of the Joint Commission on the Accreditation of Healthcare Organizations (JCAHO), was established. In the 1950s, the JCAH attempted to implement certain basic auditing procedures, but this did not prove useful. In 1966, the Medicare and Medicaid programs became effective, making it mandatory for hospitals to perform utilization review functions.

Utilization review is the process designed to monitor the need for patient admission to the hospital, the continued stay of each inpatient, and for various tests and procedures to be performed. In 1972, partly as an attempt to control spiraling health care costs, Congress passed a Social Security amendment called Public Law 92-603. This legislation mandated professional standards review organizations (PSROs). With PSRO legislation, a nationwide network of locally based physician groups was created to review the necessity, the quality, and the appropriateness of hospital care provided under the provisions of the Social Security Act.

Also in 1972, the American Hospital Association (AHA) sponsored a quality improvement program called the Quality Assurance Program for Medical Care in the Hospital as the principal framework for monitoring quality improvement in hospitals. The QIP envisioned two working committees: a utilization review committee (UR) and a medical audit committee (MA). The utilization review committee had five separate elements: 1) the certification of admission, 2) preadmission testing, 3) length of stay (LOS) certification, 4) length of stay review, and 5) discharge planning. The medical audit phase of the program stressed development of objective criteria and provided for detailed medical audits to be processed and measured against those criteria.

HOSPITAL COMMITTEES TO ADVANCE QUALITY

The hospital has continued to use quality control mechanisms primarily through its committee structure of medical staff organization. These classic control mechanisms stemmed from medical staff bylaws, rules, and regulations, and drew their authority from the board of trustees. Among major quality control mechanisms that should be in each medical staff's bylaws is a committee structure that includes: 1) a medical records committee to review contents, appropriateness, and timeliness of medical records; 2) a medical audit committee designed to conduct studies of clinical problems and practices; and 3) a utilization review committee responsible for monitoring length of stay and other utilization review activities.

Additionally, a medical staff morbidity and mortality committee will review unusual deaths and watch for patterns of death. The infection control committee of the medical staff handles episodes of hospital-acquired infections and other infectious outbreaks. The tissue committee is another important committee that exercises control over quality. It is charged with the responsibility of studying and examining tissue removed through surgical procedures. It submits its reports to the medical staff executive committee.

The credentials committee is charged with the responsibility of interviewing and reviewing credentials and recommending privileges (or denial of privileges) for each new medical staff candidate. There may be a hospital risk management department (discussed later in chapter 21, and which is much different than the safety department, which is discussed in chapter 22) whose responsibility is to monitor incidents that could result in liability suits, to analyze suits, and to establish preventive actions. Many hospitals have a pharmacy and therapeutics committee for monitoring prescribing practices, for assessing questionable prescribing of new drugs, and for considering new drugs for the formulary.

Newer Approaches

For quality improvement to be performed properly, it must be integrated with a utilization review (UR). As previously mentioned, utilization review is a means for reviewing the appropriateness, necessity, and quality of care provided during a patient's hospitalization. A review may be done prior to or following treatment, in the form of a preadmission review or a retrospective review. The UR function has been largely driven by DRGs and capitation agreements and various regulatory programs. Professional (peer) review organizations (PROs) mandated with the Medicare program replaced professional standards review (PSRO) in 1986. The PRO have more recently become Quality Improvement Organization (QIO) to better reflect its function. These organizations ensure that services provided to

Medicare beneficiaries are necessary and appropriate. The QIOs employ nurses who perform utilization reviews on federally financed patient care in hospitals. The nurse reviewer may be employed by a hospital that has been given reviewer responsibility from the QIOs. The government has let QIOs take the lead in evaluating quality improvement.

Clinical outcomes have become an important tool for hospitals to increase quality. Measuring outcomes involves examining the process, or that which is done, as well as the outcome, or the results of care. There is a strong focus on the patient and in understanding which treatments do and do not contribute to patient care.

There have been external pressures from federal and state governments to monitor and improve health care quality. The Centers for Medicare and Medicaid Services (CMS) (previously called Health Care Financing Administration) has begun to publish hospital mortality and morbidity rates each year. CMS has found a significant correlation between high mortality rates and quality problems.

In 1987, the Joint Commission mandated several steps to modernize accreditation. A key component was the integration of performance measurement into the accreditation process using the ORYX initiative. ORYX is a quality improvement plan that requires US hospitals to select (from a group of JCAHO-approved vendors) two or more clinical performance measures that relate to at least 20 percent of the patient population. The vendor will then report on behalf of the institution. The hospital selects indicators that will measure performance (defined as what is done and how well it is done). These will be reported and will 1) provide a comparison of care from hospital to hospital, 2) allow a hospital to establish a baseline to track improvement, 3) provide accountability to the public, and 4) allow external stakeholders to make decisions concerning which hospital to contract with for quality health care. The JCAHO began publishing organization-specific performance data in July 2004, allowing institutions to measure themselves against other institutions that selected the same indicators. This service became available for the public to view during January 2005 at http://www.medicare.gov.

Defining Audit Terms

The medical audit is one of the principal tools used to evaluate quality care in institutions. It is necessary to clearly understand definitions used in the medical audit process. There are at least three generally accepted systems used in conducting a medical audit: the structure system, the process system, and the outcome system.

The structure system is one in which the hospital and its medical staff evaluate the setting in which care is provided and resources are made available to the physician and practitioner. This system deals primarily with the adequacy of the hospital's facilities and work force.

A process audit refers to what the physician actually does to diagnose and treat the patient. This involves the source of medical care and the patient's compliance with the physician's orders.

An outcome audit concerns the actual results of the care given. Questions should address the outcome of the treatment. For example, did the patient respond properly to treatment? What was the mortality rate for treatment? Was the patient able to perform regular daily activities? Did the patient have any psychological effects?

Because there are three kinds of structures, or systems, for evaluation, the hospital has the opportunity to review quality while the patient is in the hospital and retrospectively in terms of what happened after the patient left the hospital, based on the patient's medical record. In traditional medical audits, hospitals usually include a retrospective review of the medical care process, based on the patient's medical record. More recently, questions of outcome and patient satisfaction are also being considered.

Although the principal function of a medical audit should be to improve patient care, there are also byproducts. Deficiencies are noted and can be corrected, thus improving patient care. A byproduct would be that the audit method encourages coordination of physicians with other health team members in patient care planning. Also, documentation of patient care is improved through medical records. Additional direction is given to continuing education for physicians and health care personnel. The need for new equipment or facilities can be brought to the attention of hospital management. Finally, a proper medical audit may provide written documentation to the board of trustees, showing the status of medical care as practiced within certain diagnoses in the hospital.

The Board's Responsibility

In a landmark legal suit in 1965, *Darling v. Charleston Community Hospital,*[1] the court ruled that a hospital and its board of trustees must assume shared responsibility for medical care of patients in the hospital. Other court interpretations have confirmed the hospital's obligation to oversee the medical staff in the quality of care. The board of trustees should play a role in the hospital's structuring of quality control systems. It must make sure that the medical staff is well organized and that appropriate and effective medical audit procedures are implemented in the hospital.

Automated Quality Improvement

The computer software industry has developed information systems to monitor the severity of inpatient illnesses. These systems are capable of collecting patient care data, computing the data against standards, and interpreting the results. Hospitals are better able to assess the patient on admission, at peak clinical severity, and at discharge with this automated information. Quality problems such as an inappropriate percentage of deaths at a certain level of severity can be identified. Hospitals using computerized information may be able to respond better to demands made by regulators involving the submission of severity, morbidity, and mortality reports.

The Future of Quality Improvement

As described in the Newer Approaches section, hospitals will be increasingly in the spotlight to report outcomes. As consumers become better informed, they will seek out institutions providing the best outcomes. Hospitals will increasingly use balanced scorecards (a simplistic method of reporting key indicators) to report quality improvement performance; the results may be reported publicly.

CHAPTER REVIEW

1. What is quality improvement and why is it so important in a hospital?
2. What is utilization review?
3. What is the function of the mortality and morbidity committee?
4. What is CMS, and what did it replace?
5. What is ORYX?
6. What is the board's role in quality improvement?
7. What is the role of the tissue committee?
8. Define clinical indicators and clinical outcomes.
9. What is the function of the credentials committee? List at least six items that it would want to examine in an application for privileges.
10. Discuss the Leapfrog organization and what it is doing to improve quality and outcomes in health care.

NOTE

1. *Darling v. Charleston Community Hospital*, 211 N.E. 2d 253 (1965) cert. denied 383 V.S. 946.

Chapter 21

Risk Management and Medical Malpractice

Key Terms

Damages

Defensive medicine

Incident report

Loss prevention

Malpractice

Negligence

Plaintiff

Respondent superior

Risk manager

RISK MANAGEMENT

Risk management is an early warning system for identifying potential causes of liability and for averting their occurrences. The primary function of risk management is to coordinate and implement loss prevention and corrective activities throughout the hospital. Another way of saying this is to reduce the hospital's liability—liabilities from patients, visitors, and employees. An added function is to receive, evaluate, and maintain confidential reports on incidents and/or accidents occurring in the institution. The incident report is the primary instrument used to provide clues identifying a risk situation.

RISK MANAGEMENT AS A TEAM APPROACH

Though an individual is designated as the hospital's risk manager (the person charged with examining areas of risk of liability and then working to minimize this risk), a team approach is essential for effective risk management. In addition to the risk manager, team members include administrators, members of the governing body, physicians, professional staff, the in-house attorney (if the hospital employs one), other employees, a retained lawyer from the community, and possibly insurance consultants.

Risk management should be integrated with the hospital's traditional quality improvement committees—utilization review, quality improvement, safety and loss control, and infection control.

RISK MANAGEMENT AND QUALITY IMPROVEMENT

Even though risk management and quality improvement are individual practices with independent functions, some of these functions overlap. For instance, the primary purpose of risk management is to protect the hospital's assets, whereas the fundamental reason for quality improvement is to protect patients. The primary duty in risk management is to identify all risk exposures, whereas in quality improvement it is to measure care against standards. Risk management is apt to be a prospective activity; quality improvement is largely a retrospective activity.

MEDICAL MALPRACTICE

Risk management has proven to be a beneficial tool for hospitals in the prevention of medical malpractice suits.[1] Detecting substandard practices and correcting them prevents malpractice claims. Discussing occurrences with patients and families can further discourage litigation. Risk management also helps to ensure that physicians and health care professionals are practicing according to acceptable standards.

Overview of Malpractice (Tort Law)

The phenomenon of malpractice that began to flourish in the early 1960s has continued to grow in the health care field. In 1973, medical malpractice was defined in a complete study by the Department of Health, Education, and Welfare. The department's *Report of the Secretary's Commission on Malpractice* stated:

> Medical malpractice has been defined as an injury to a patient caused by a health care provider's negligence; a malpractice claim is an allegation with or without foundation that an injury was caused by negligence; injury implies either physical or mental harm that occurs in the course of medical care whether or not it is caused by negligence; compensation requires proof of both an injury and professional negligence.[2]

A tort is a legal term meaning a civil wrong or harm for which the remedy is the awarding of money to compensate the victim for the damages incurred.

Medical malpractice cases allege breaches of tort law. To win a malpractice suit, the plaintiff (the individual suing the hospital) must meet four standards. First, the plaintiff must prove that the provider of care (the physician or hospital) owed a duty to the patient, for example, to do no harm; second, that the duty was breached (harm was done); third, the plaintiff must show that he or she incurred damages of some sort; and fourth, that the damages resulted directly from the breach.

DEFENSIVE MEDICINE

Although only an estimated 3 to 8 percent of physicians are sued annually as a direct result of medical malpractice, there has been an alarming increase in defensive medicine practiced by physicians. Defensive medicine is generally thought of as unnecessary tests or procedures done to ward off lawsuits. The costs for additional tests performed to protect the physician are staggering.

HOSPITAL LIABILITY FOR PHYSICIANS' ACTS

It is important to recognize that in some cases a hospital may be held liable for physicians' negligent acts. The most frequent occasion for this is when the hospital permits an incompetent or unqualified physician to treat a patient. The hospital can be held liable even when the physician is not employed by the hospital. The institution is not held liable for the negligent act that caused harm to the patient, but it is held liable for its own negligence in permitting the physician to treat the patient. Attorneys argue that a physician's incompetence should be known to hospital authorities. These are generally negligent credentialing cases whereby the hospital granted privileges to an incompetent physician or allowed one to practice while under the influence of drugs or alcohol.

RESPONDENT SUPERIOR

Under the doctrine of *respondent superior*, "the master is liable for the actions of the servant," the traditional thought is of the employer (hospital) being sued if the employee harms a patient, visitor, or guest. However, the courts have expanded this to include apparent employees. For example, if a *contract* physician who is *not* a hospital employee is working in the emergency department and harms a patient, the patient may sue the physician *and* the hospital if the physician *appears* to be an employee. Hospitals can remove the apparent problem by requiring emergency department nonemployee physicians to wear name tags with their company names (such as "1st Rate Emergency Physician," Dr. Thomas) and posting signs in the emergency department stating that the physicians on duty are a contract group and are not hospital employees.

ROLE OF THE MEDICAL RECORD

It may be up to 2 years after an incident occurs before a hospital administrator or physician receives a notice of suit. When this happens, the first step is for the physician or administrator to request the patient's medical record. The hospital medical record should depict, in written fashion, the course of the patient's care and treatment while in the hospital. The record is the medium of communication among members of the hospital health team. It is also frequently a factor in whether a plaintiff wins the case. Juries and malpractice lawyers are not likely to accept reasoning that the chart was not written clearly enough at the time. The medical record must accurately reflect the true events of hospitalization; there is no substitute for good documentation in winning a malpractice lawsuit.

When an administrator receives a suit against the hospital, the physician is frequently named as well. It is a good procedure to make a copy of the medical record for the hospital's attorney as well as for the physician's attorney. The original medical record should be placed under lock and key in the medical records department while the case is in litigation.

CHAPTER REVIEW

1. What is the function of the risk manager?
2. What are four necessary elements of a medical malpractice case?
3. What is the doctrine of *respondent superior*?
4. What is medical malpractice?
5. What is the difference between risk management and quality improvement?
6. What is defensive medicine?
7. What is a tort? Is it a form of civil law or criminal law?
8. Define "intentional tort" and list several examples. How are intentional torts different from negligence? Are both intentional torts and negligence actions found in medicine? If so, give examples.

NOTES

1. For further discussion of health care law, please see Pozgar, George, *Legal Aspects of Health Care Administration*, 9th ed., Sudbury, MA: Jones and Bartlett Publishers, 2004.
2. US Department of Health, Education, and Welfare, 1973, *Report of the Secretary's Commission on Medical Malpractice*, Department of Health, Education and Welfare publication no. (08) 73–88, 1973, p. 4.

Chapter 22

Patient Safety

THE PROBLEM OF MEDICAL ERRORS

A report by the Institute of Medicine, a nongovernmental Washington, D.C. think tank, estimates that in the United States, between 44,000 and 98,000 people die each year of preventable medical errors such as drug interactions. This makes medical mistakes the eighth leading cause of death in the United States, ahead of AIDS, breast cancer, and car wrecks.[1]

During the Clinton presidency, the Advisory Commission on Consumer Protection and Quality in the Health Care Industry reported a much higher number. According to the commission's 1998 report, perhaps as many as 180,000 die from errors and medical mishaps.[2]

Errors involving contraindications (directives for drugs that shouldn't be given to a particular patient, sometimes because the patient is pregnant, is allergic to the drug, or is engaged in certain activities such as operating heavy machinery) or interactions (directives that certain medications should not be taken with each other, or with certain foods) can occur when drugs are prescribed or when they are administered, such as drugs being given to the wrong patient, at the wrong time, or in the wrong dose. Still other errors occur when someone incorrectly transcribes the name or dose of the drug, perhaps because they cannot read the physician's handwriting. Yet other errors take place when the medication drip is incorrectly administered.

ENDING MEDICAL ERRORS

Errors do not have to happen. Simple acts such as one nurse preparing the medication and another nurse checking it will stop many problems. Storage of heparin and insulin (which are similar in appearance) in different areas will eliminate many administration mistakes.

It is estimated that the use of computers in health care could eliminate as many as two million drug interactions and 190,000 hospitalizations each year.[3] An additional study suggests that 86% of medication errors could be removed through ordering drugs electronically.[4] This would eliminate problems of bad handwriting, errors of reading and switching similar-appearing medication names, and the too-frequent problem of misunderstanding medication pronunciations.

Even without computers, some medication errors can be eliminated or reduced through better training of caregivers. For example, if caregivers are taught to use a zero before any number less than one (0.5 instead of .5) there will be less chance for error—the same is true of never using a zero after a number greater than one (2, *not* 2.0). When writing orders, print rather than script will lessen the chance for mistakes.

Other problems in the ordering and using of medications are the involvement of different caregivers and the number of steps taken when medications are prescribed. A physician writes the order, the pharmacy fills the prescription, and nurses administer the medication; in many hospitals, there are approximately twenty steps in the process. If a physician would type the medication name, dose amount, frequency of administration, and duration, many medication errors that could occur during this lengthy process would be eliminated.

Adverse drug reactions (much different from medication errors) can stem from errors such as overdosing the patient, or interactions between medications. Adverse reactions also include side effects. The use of computer software in the pharmacy could eliminate these problems; the computer is programmed to alert the pharmacist and physician as to when drug reactions could take place.

Newly approved medications or the "off-label" use of medications (the use of medications in a manner not originally intended by the drug manufacturer) can also cause problems. Many drugs taken off the market are removed in the first year of their use. Physicians must become familiar with new medications and promptly report any unusual side effects not stated by the drug manufacturers. Physicians may submit a risk form to the Food and Drug Administration, or, most often, they report directly to the pharmaceutical company.

Nurses must take care at all times. For example, suppose Patient A asks to transfer to another room because Patient B is snoring loudly. Sometime during the night, Patient C is admitted into Patient A's original room. The nurses change shift at 7:00 a.m. and the medication nurse walks in and administers insulin to Patient

C, not knowing that Patient A was moved and believing Patient C is Patient A. Insulin could be fatal if given to a nondiabetic patient. Many hospital systems are experimenting with bar-coded wrist bands that must be swiped by a wand connected to a laptop that the nurse carries. This device would give an audible warning if the wrong patient is about to get the wrong medicine.

UNITED STATES VS. EUROPEAN OPERATING ROOMS

Another area of concern regarding patient safety is surgery. Most European operating rooms (ORs) tend to be larger than ORs in the United States, often by about 100 square feet, allowing much more room for the surgery team to maneuver. These larger rooms also have space to accommodate induction and early recovery. It is anticipated that all surgery rooms of the future will have monitors and cameras that may be viewed by all members of the surgery team and operated remotely, if necessary. It is anticipated that many of the cables that now clutter the room will be eliminated by wireless technology. Surface-to-surface transfers will be eliminated by the operating room table serving as a combination transporter and tabletop. This has been available for 30 years and is popular in Europe, but not often seen in the United States. As US hospitals renovate, surgery suites likely will be updated. Another innovation for patient safety will be bar-coded or radio frequency armbands, which allow alarms to sound if the wrong patient is brought into surgery. To prevent the wrong surgery being done, many hospitals now require the surgeon to sign his name with a felt-tip pen on the actual area of the body he is about to operate on. This heightens awareness on the surgeon and operating room crew.

JCAHO

The Joint Commission on Accreditation of Health Care Organizations has mandated that institutions address and demonstrate what they are doing to improve in the seven national patient safety goals in order to participate in the JCAHO accreditation program. The seven goals are:

1. Improve the effectiveness of communication among caregivers.
2. Improve the safety of using high-alert medications.
3. Improve the safety of using infusion pumps.
4. Improve the effectiveness of clinical alarm systems.
5. Improve the accuracy of patient identification.
6. Eliminate wrong site, wrong patient, and wrong procedure surgery.
7. Reduce the risk of health care-acquired infections.

We have touched only on a very small number of patient safety areas and the reduction of some errors. Countless safety practices serve to demonstrate patient safety and are a team effort involving every department in the hospital. These practices include medical staff credentialing to insure physicians are qualified for privileges, human resources to conduct random drug screens and criminal background checks of every employee, and education and training to insure caregivers are competent in the latest clinical techniques. In addition, hospitals should implement infant security measures to minimize the risk of abductions; infection control measures to minimize hospital-acquired infections; and surgery procedures including providing informed consent forms, confirming the correct patient, site, and procedure, and ensuring the surgeon is competent to perform the procedure.

Zero tolerance for errors and unsafe practices should be the goal of every health care institution.

CHAPTER REVIEW

1. Where do medical mistakes rank in the list of leading causes of death in the United States?
2. What are medication errors? Give five examples.
3. What are adverse drug reactions? Give three examples.
4. Discuss how medication errors may be prevented.
5. What are the seven National Patient Safety Goals mandated in the JCAHO accreditation program?
6. How can computers be used to reduce medical errors? Discuss pharmacy software that is specifically designed for this purpose.
7. What are off-label uses of medication and why is this practice sometimes dangerous?
8. How can bar-coding be used to reduce patient errors?
9. Discuss how nosocomial (hospital-acquired) infections can be reduced. Should the infection control nurse be part of the nursing department or the quality improvement department?

NOTES

1. "Healthcare's Outrageous IT Gap," *The Economist*, April 30–May 6th, 2005, pp. 61–63.
2. The White House, Office of the Press Secretary, "Establishment of the Quality Interagency Coordination Task Force," March 13, 1998.
3. *The Economist*, 2005.
4. *The Economist*, 2005.

Chapter 23

Bioethics

INTRODUCTION

As medicine advances, society is impacted continually with new decisions regarding beginning of life and end of life issues. We save premature babies with success, and we keep patients alive much longer. Society must have a framework with which to make intelligent decisions regarding these issues. The theories and issues involved in establishing this framework are known as bioethics. Ethics is an area of philosophy that deals with understanding and examining morals, as in "knowing the difference between right and wrong." Bioethics is often described as ethics applied to life. The question of "what is right and what is wrong" is open to intense debate; issues include but are not limited to abortion, physician-assisted suicide, distributing limited resources such as kidneys and livers, and a host of other medical issues.

Hospitals and physicians are often called upon to assist family decision makers. Most hospitals have a bioethics committee or panel that may be convened quickly. This voluntary committee is usually comprised of at least one physician, nurse, social worker, administrator, and a member of the community clergy; each has usually received some training in bioethics. Committee members often carry beepers and can be telephoned or summoned to meet and discuss a pending case and then give suggestions, recommendations, or guidelines to those who have elicited the help of the committee. Other hospitals employ a single clinical ethicist to provide consultations or to be a resource person. The background of these people can be religious studies, medicine, law, or philosophy.

To guide the committee, or for that matter, family members or physicians, the field of bioethics utilizes four primary pillars, although there are more. The primary pillars are autonomy, nonmaleficence, beneficence, and social justice.

THE PRINCIPLE OF AUTONOMY

In the recent past, patients usually followed the advice of their physician. These learned medical professionals could instruct or order the patient to take a course of action and would expect the patient to follow the instructed course. As patients have become more enlightened and educated, many now want and expect to make their own medical decisions, hence the discussion of autonomy. These patients want all options presented, but then would like to undertake the decision themselves. The medical profession is learning to grant or respect the wishes of the patient, allowing the patient to be autonomous.

This rather simple notion becomes a bit more complex as we explore it. What if the patient is incapacitated or otherwise unable to undertake his own medical decisions; e.g., in cases of dementia, coma, or involving a minor? What if there are factors that coerce a patient to decide for or against a particular course of treatment . . . is her decision truly voluntary? Therefore, we add stipulations to that autonomy—the decision the patient is making must be voluntary, with understanding of the consequences, without controlling influences, and the patient must have the mental capacity to decide.

In the area of autonomy, it should be noted that before surgery or other procedures are performed, an informed consent form is presented to the patient for signature. This helps to protect the patient by stating in writing what could occur, and it protects the hospital and caregivers by demonstrating that the patient was informed and that the procedure was undertaken freely.

A troubling area for some regarding autonomy is when a patient wishes to undertake a course of action not in agreement with others. For example, when it is the autonomous wish of a quadriplegic patient to discontinue feeding and hydration, should the hospital grant this wish, knowing the consequence? The courts will usually side with the patient's wishes.

Is autonomy always granted? After all, doesn't each person own one's own body? Autonomy is not an absolute right. For example, courts have ruled that while we may sell plasma or women may sell their eggs, we may not sell kidneys or other organs due to the doctrine that this is against public interest.

THE PRINCIPLE OF NONMALEFICENCE

The principle of nonmaleficence was discussed by Hippocrates when he said, "First, do no harm." This is understood to mean to do no harm either by acts of commission or omission. For example, it is understood not to administer the wrong medication to the patient, and it is understood that the necessary medicines must be properly administered without missing a prescribed dose. If one imposes unreasonable or careless risks of harm to a patient, the caregivers may find themselves facing a negligence medical malpractice lawsuit.

In further exploring nonmaleficence, we find that this principle embraces medical competence. Physicians are now held to a nationwide standard rather than a community standard as was common in the recent past. There is a different standard for diverse board certification; surgeons are held to a higher standard than a general practitioner is if both are performing the same surgical procedure.

THE PRINCIPLE OF BENEFICENCE

Besides the principle of nonmaleficence, there is an added duty that benefits the patient. This means not only acting in the patient's best interest, but also entails taking the extra step to protect the patient and remove harm.

What constitutes the patient's best interest? What if the patient is elderly and has a terminal disease . . . should he be resuscitated if he goes into cardiac arrest? Is this truly benefiting him? Advanced directives (forms that will assist caregivers in understanding what an incapacitated patient would decide if the patient had the capacity to make the decision) become important in these instances to allow caregivers to better make a decision that reflects the patient's wishes.

THE PRINCIPLE OF SOCIAL JUSTICE

As a society, we wish to be fair, and being fair means having a uniform manner for distributing resources. We understand that goods and services will always be limited; therefore, we must try to allocate societal assets like health care in an equitable way. It is generally agreed that equal beings should receive equal treatment, but it is also agreed that while everyone would like to drive a Porsche, society can only afford to provide buses. This is where the principle of social justice must be considered. Social justice involves the fair distribution of scarce resources. But what is fair is often debated.

Consequently, what should be the distribution of scarce resources? Should we distribute resources according to peoples' needs? Should everyone receive an equal share? If the answer is yes, and there are four patients awaiting a liver transplant, should each get one fourth? What if thirty-seven patients are waiting? This will not work because they all need the complete liver. Other methods that could be discussed to determine who gets the liver are:

- "To each patient according to his or her merit?" Is a teacher more valuable to society than a bank teller or a dog trainer more valuable than a police officer? Who determines merit?
- "To each patient according to his or her ability to pay?" This hardly seems fair, due to the many who seek employment so they can benefit society without seeking a large salary, e.g., clergy, teachers, etc. In addition, many people view health care as a right.
- "To each patient by a random lottery?" In this case, all patients could enter their Social Security numbers in a drawing; one winner gets the needed resource. This might seem fair unless we discover that the liver winner was an alcoholic and had self-inflicted her own disease. Is it fair to allocate the liver to her, rather than to someone who has never touched alcohol?
- "To each patient based on life expectancy?" Should a 10-year-old girl with her whole life ahead of her take precedence over someone who has already lived a full life? Should we make age the criteria with the youngest always getting the resource? Would it surprise you to learn that several countries allocate health care in a similar manner; those above a certain age do not qualify for a state-sponsored procedure (but they may still have the procedure if they have adequate private resources to pay for it).

Perhaps the answer to the social justice dilemma in the United States is to have universal health care with everyone entitled to a minimum, basic, and decent standard of health care; above this level, society members would have to purchase added care (plastic surgery, orthodontics, laser assisted in situ keratomileusis [LASIK] eye surgery, etc.).

A FINAL WORD

Bioethics is a segment of philosophy that may often find itself embroiled in conflict; there may often be deep-seeded disagreement among caregivers, patients, and their family members. The role of the hospital bioethics committee is to lend gentle advice when it is sought, and to present topics that may not have occurred to those less objective and who could be very emotional because of their proximity to the issues. The cases of Karen Ann Quinlan, Nancy Cruzan, and Terri Schiavo (comatose patients who were in persistive vegetative states) were fought in the courts for years, possibly because of paternalistic interests of those who wished to override the patient's wishes. The role of the bioethics committee is to suggest ways to safeguard the patient's wishes and rights.

CHAPTER REVIEW

1. What is bioethics?
2. Who is usually invited or appointed to the bioethics committee?
3. What is autonomy?
4. What is nonmaleficence?
5. What is beneficence?
6. What is social justice?

DISCUSSION QUESTIONS

1. What is ethics?
2. Discuss this statement: Bioethics does not often have answers to which everyone agrees.
3. Discuss the bioethical problems (if any) with transplanting a face, as was first done in December 2005.
4. Are bioethical issues universal among people and nations? For example, your hospital has a Muslim patient who is in need of a bioethics consultation. Should the bioethics committee consult with a religious leader within the local Muslim community and invite him or her to attend the meeting to give advice?
5. In December 1991, hospitals participating in Medicare and Medicaid were required to inform their patients of their right to "self-determination" as it corresponds to their existing state law. Research and report on your state's law regarding "durable power of attorney for healthcare decisions" and "advanced directives."

Chapter 24

Accreditation and Licensing

HISTORICAL REVIEW

How do patients and community residents know whether the hospital in their community, or the hospital they are unfortunate enough to be in as a patient is a good hospital? How does a patient know if an outside organization has reviewed the systems, the procedures, the physicians, nurses, and all else in the hospital to make sure it is all working properly? Fortunately, a group whose sole purpose is to review hospitals exists. It then informs hospitals, patients, and the community whether a hospital is satisfactory. This process of review is called hospital accreditation, and the group that undertakes this is called the Joint Commission on Accreditation of Healthcare Organizations (JCAHO), formerly known as the Joint Commission on Accreditation of Hospitals (JCAH).

The JCAHO traced its roots to a program called the Hospital Standardization Program that the American College of Surgeons established in 1918. The college established the program to enable surgeons to understand and appreciate the uniform medical records format that would allow them to evaluate members who wished to apply for fellowship status in the American College of Surgeons. From this beginning, the group joined with three other groups—the American College of Physicians, the American Medical Association, and the American Hospital Association—to form the JCAH. On January 1, 1952, the Joint Commission officially began its work of surveying hospitals and granting accreditation. After its first year, it was clear that it had to have a more dynamic nature, and its standards were amended slightly. Ever since then, the Joint Commission has done a credible job of keeping up with new standards in the United States and constantly revising its approach to those standards. In the early years of the Joint Commission, up until 1961, field studies were done by member organizations that were part of the JCAH. In 1961, the Joint Commission hired its own full-time field staff.

In 1964, the Joint Commission began to charge a survey fee to hospitals in order to complete its field program. With the passage of Medicare legislation, Public Law 89-97 in 1965, the Joint Commission was given a necessary boost. It was written into the Medicare Act that hospitals participating under Medicare had to meet a certain level of quality of patient care as measured against a recognized norm. The JCAHO was specifically referred to in the law and hospitals were told they could undergo either a Medicare survey or a JCAHO survey. This was reaffirmed by the Social Security Administration in its standards of 1965.

While the JCAHO introduced medical audit requirements in the early 1970s, it also adopted broad requirements concerning the review and evaluation of the quality and appropriateness of health care. In 1979, the JCAHO developed new standards that required hospitals to develop quality improvement programs according to the quality assessment activities required by JCAHO standards. The Joint Commission has since adopted this standard for all other types of health care organizations that it accredits, and JCAHO's focus has essentially become quality improvement. The change of name from the Joint Commission on Accreditation of Hospitals to Joint Commission of Healthcare Organizations that occurred in September 1987 more accurately reflects its mission and the constituencies it serves. Today, JCAHO often surveys home health agencies, hospice care, and other types of health care providers.

During the 1980s, JCAHO became more involved in the use of information systems. It now uses a computerized system in its survey analysis process. The Joint Commission also has a database that can help explain variations in outcomes of hospital care. The database represents a potential use of performance data to improve quality of care.

ACCREDITATION OVERVIEW

How does a hospital become accredited? The hospital completes an application and asks the JCAHO, located in Chicago, to survey the hospital. The Joint Commission sends to the hospital a large, complex, comprehensive questionnaire that addresses standards for a hospital. After the hospital has completed the questionnaire and returned it, a survey team is assigned by JCAHO and a date is selected for a site visit to the hospital.

The questionnaire, and therefore the standards, are concerned with three major areas:

1. *The services and quality of services the hospital delivers to the patient.* The JCAHO reviews the medical staff organization and systems, nursing, dietary services, the pharmacy, respiratory care, imaging, physical therapy, emergency department services, etc. It determines whether services provided are adequate for patients. It is important to note that laboratories are surveyed by their own association, that of the College of American Pathologists (CAP). Both the Joint Commission and Medicare recognize this in lieu of conducting their own survey.

2. *The principles of organization and administration.* Does the hospital have an effective bylaws structure? Does it have written policies and procedures? Does it require its departments to meet on a regular basis and to present written reports? Is the board involved and does it provide adequate oversight?

3. *The physical plant and the environment in the hospital.* This includes life-safety code problems, whether the hospital has adequate sprinkler systems, whether the corridors are large enough, whether there are proper safety exits, etc.

Recently, the Joint Commission has been spending a great deal of time and effort on quality improvement reviews in patient care areas. The surveyors review patient medical records and other reports to determine whether care given is appropriate for a specific case.

The Joint Commission publishes a reference manual for hospitals called the Accreditation Manual for Hospitals (AMH). This manual contains the standards used by the Joint Commission to evaluate hospitals. The reader is cautioned that the JCAHO periodically changes its standards to maintain best practices for hospitals. It is imperative that the hospital to be surveyed is current on the latest survey standards.

ACCREDITATION IN MORE DETAIL

After the hospital completes the survey and the questionnaire, a JCAHO survey team is scheduled to visit the hospital. The JCAHO survey team consists of a physician, a nurse, and sometimes a hospital administrator. If it is a large hospital, the survey team may consist of three members and usually takes 3 to 4 days to complete the survey. If it is a very small hospital, there may be two members (a physician and a nurse) and the survey may involve only a 2- to 3-day visit.

The survey is quite complete and well organized. Each member of the survey team has a specific area to observe and survey. During the survey, which is actually a walk-through of the hospital, the surveyors read procedure manuals and minutes of meetings, look at life-safety code issues such as smoke barriers and sprinkler systems, examine crash carts to ensure they are periodically inventoried and inspected at the change of each nursing shift, interview personnel, and note any deficiencies observed in the hospital. They then make recommendations. Before they leave the hospital, they give their list to the hospital administrator at a formal exit briefing. The survey team reviews with the administrator and key members of the administrator's staff exactly what they found in need of improvement and what they recommend. This is a very open, candid discussion on how the hospital can improve itself. The surveyors send their list and reports to JCAHO headquarters, where they are reviewed in detail. Finally, the JCAHO makes a decision, based upon the survey, whether the hospital should be accredited. Though many hospitals receive accreditation from the JCAHO, there are different modifiers to the accreditation; e.g., accreditation with commendation, accredited, or conditionally accredited.

After a hospital has been accredited by the JCAHO, it receives a certificate of accreditation indicating this achievement. If it receives a three-year accreditation, it must, in the interim period before the next JCAHO visit, complete a detailed questionnaire identifying what was done to correct the deficiencies noted in the original survey. The interim questionnaire is sent to the Joint Commission in Chicago where it is evaluated.

The JCAHO is important in the evaluation of hospitals in the United States. It is unique because it is voluntary. The JCAHO has been responsive to hospitals and the state and federal government. It provides a silent service to the patient and community; it maintains high professional standards; it acts as an advisory group to hospitals and is influential in urging hospitals to improve their life-safety measures, their quality improvement programs, and their organizations.

WHAT DOES ACCREDITATION REALLY MEAN TO A HOSPITAL?

The hospital that has become accredited says to its community, its patients, and staff that it wants to meet high standards and that it has exerted the effort and time to have the Joint Commission measure it against a set standard. Accreditation tells a hospital's employees and patients that the environment is of high quality and personnel are qualified to provide care. Accreditation emphasizes that the hospital is a responsible institution that takes its obligations for patient care seriously and has asked an independent, objective group to review it.

SENTINEL EVENTS

The Joint Commission requires health care organizations to report sentinel events, which are defined as unexpected occurrences involving death, serious physical or psychological injury, or the risk thereof. This includes unanticipated death or major permanent loss of function not related to a patient's illness. It also includes events such as surgery on the wrong patient or body part, infant abductions, patients who commit suicide or are raped while in the hospital, or transfusion reactions caused by major blood group incompatibilities.

After reporting a sentinel event, the organization should conduct a root cause analysis to uncover the basic factor(s) that led to the problem. This should assist the organization in enhancing their performance outcomes and avoiding similar problems. In addition to the thorough investigation, the organization should seek "best practices" (as defined in the current literature and the seminars held by professional groups) and make changes to reduce future instances. They should identify who will be responsible for necessary changes, set a time line for the changes, educate the staff regarding the change, and then implement and monitor the changes, evaluating the effectiveness of the change.

JOINT COMMISSION INTERNATIONAL

As the reader has learned in other parts of this text, many hospitals voluntarily undertake an accreditation survey from the Joint Commission on Accreditation of Healthcare Organizations in order to 1) receive federal funding, 2) demonstrate to the public that they are a quality institution, or 3) to improve their own internal processes.

Hospitals outside the United States have wanted a similar accreditation process so that they may demonstrate quality and thus attract patients and physicians. In 1999, the Joint Commission announced standards for international hospitals under the name Joint Commission International (JCI). Hospitals outside the United States may apply for an accreditation survey, prepare for the survey, and then receive a site visit from a survey team. The accreditation visit is conducted in a similar manner to that of one in the United States.

LICENSURE

The JCAHO reviews and surveys are the primary controls over hospitals. In fact, the accreditation is somewhat like an informal license, particularly since the federal government, under Titles XVIII and XIX of the Medicare legislation, Public Law 89-97, has endorsed the Joint Commission's survey in order to certify payment for hospitals under Medicare legislation. There are other forms of control working in the hospital system as well.

Formal licensing is the most common form of regulation by the states. Generally, a license to operate a hospital is issued by a state agency, perhaps the health department. The licensing bureau or agency can retain records of a hospital's bed capacity and the capabilities of its other facilities. The states' health and welfare departments account for three quarters of the state agencies that have regulatory powers over hospitals. A state's licensure laws and regulations usually culminate in a licensure inspection that is similar to the inspection conducted by the JCAHO. This accounts for one of the overlaps in the regulatory system. Frequently, state and Joint Commission inspectors inspect the same things, or the state will accept the JCAHO accreditation process and not conduct an inspection.

The JCAHO reciprocally shares survey information with state and district licensure agencies regarding a hospital's accreditation surveys. In turn, these agencies report information about potential standard-related problems in accredited hospitals to the Joint Commission. Reciprocally sharing information enables both the Joint Commission and licensure agencies to identify hospitals that have performance problems, and as a result, require further review.

MEDICARE CERTIFICATION

Another form of control used for hospitals beyond licensure is the process of Medicare certification. Hospitals must be certified since the 1965 Social Security Amendments that sponsored Titles XVIII and XIX. At that time, the federal government established a way for hospitals to participate in federal insurance programs, but indicated that they had to meet certain general compliance guidelines to do so. For example, hospitals could establish an around-the-clock nursing staff, certain medical supervision, and the proper use of clinical records. This step then led to formal Medicare surveys.

Medicare Survey

Should a hospital not wish to undertake a Joint Commission survey (usually because these are expensive, involving fees to JCAHO and considerable preparation time needed to be successful) the hospital may opt to undertake a Medicare survey. Without a successfully completed JCAHO or Medicare survey, the hospital will not qualify for Medicare funding.

REGISTRATION

Registration is a weak form of control in the system. It might not even be regarded by hospital authorities as a control. However, a system of registration exists that identifies hospitals and other health care institutions in order for third parties, consumers, and federal agencies to review the rosters of such institutions. The most common registration in the hospital system is conducted by the American Hospital Association (AHA). The AHA maintains an extensive system of data collection in the form of hospital profiles. It is also involved in registering hospitals in planning areas. For example, the AHA reviews new construction, proposed mergers, and the proposed sharing of services. The AHA publishes an annual hospital statistics report that includes data from many of its registration activities.

CHAPTER REVIEW

1. What is JCAHO?
2. Who comprises a survey team?
3. What is a recognized alternative survey to JCAHO?

DISCUSSION QUESTIONS

1. Research the hospital licensing criteria for your state, and discuss the strengths and weaknesses of the criteria.
2. What is JCI? Are the standards the same as standards for US hospitals?
3. What is a sentinel event? Can a hospital report such an event and still insulate itself against litigation? Call several healthcare attorneys in your area and report their opinions.
4. Discuss the pros and cons of undertaking a JCAHO survey as opposed to undertaking a Medicare survey.

Part IX
Continuing to Grow

Chapter 25

Hospital Marketing

INTRODUCTION

It can be argued that hospital care is something everybody needs and therefore should not have to be marketed at all. Traditionally, hospitals, like the rest of the health care field, have avoided marketing. They have resisted advertising and competitive pricing though they were willing to attempt to improve their public and community image. Yet with a finite patient population and many communities being overbedded, some hospitals have found themselves in a fierce fight for their very survival, pitted against other hospitals, pulling out all stops to maintain market share.

Marketing today is very sophisticated and is a combination of self-analysis, market research, competitor research, and demographic research, carefully noting trends and then plotting a strategy to maximize market share. It comes down to knowing who you are (*you* being the hospital), who they are (*they* being the rival hospitals), and the needs of the target population. The target population could be patients, physicians, or insurance companies . . . after all, patients don't admit themselves; hospitals have no patients unless physicians admit the patients; and many patients must visit a certain hospital based on their insurance coverage.

Marketing suggests that hospitals should try to determine both the physicians' and the community's needs, and that the strategy should attempt to meet these needs by developing appropriate services, testing, and treatment programs.

Other factors—soaring health costs, increased participation among patients in meeting their own health care needs and in selecting their providers, and higher expectations from health care consumers—have driven hospitals to increase their marketing efforts.

WHAT IS MARKETING?

Marketing is a system of activities that combines product, place, price, and promotion in order to properly distribute goods and services to the target population. In a market exchange this can be viewed as a certain individual being persuaded to give another individual something in order to receive a service, good, or privilege in return. Four of the more active areas of marketing are 1) public relations, 2) advertising, 3) research, and 4) sales.

Public Relations—Only One Part of the Marketing Effort

Public relations (PR) has been generally defined as developing an image and goodwill between the public and a person, firm, or institution.

For many years, hospitals have understood the need to develop and retain positive relationships with their patients, their potential donors, and their community at large. Public relations can improve a hospital's image, generate the public's interest, and aid in fund-raising efforts. Most hospitals probably have a somewhat formal or informal public relations program. Many have a full-time public relations staff. The main objective of this staff is to position the hospital to receive favorable publicity in the community. To accomplish this, staff might invite a local newspaper editor to tour the hospital, thereby improving the chances of favorable publicity, or it could develop strong contacts with a local television and radio station, thereby improving relationships with the media.

The public relations department is a staff or advisory department. Generally, there is a public relations director in charge of the department. The PR department works closely with all other hospital departments, but the public relations function is clearly the responsibility of hospital management. The technical aspects of public relations, such as developing brochures or writing press releases, are usually left to a technical expert. A public relations program need not necessarily be costly or elaborate, but it must be well thought out and systematically developed with managerial input if it is to be effective and get the message across in a proper manner.

A community hospital has two public relations constituents. The first is an internal public—the hospital's board of trustees, its employees, medical staff members, volunteers, patients, and friends of the hospital. This internal public is relatively easy to target and sell with the hospital's positive public image. This is usually accomplished through a series of traditional publications such as hospital newsletters.

The more difficult segment to reach is the hospital's external public. This consists of potential patients of the hospital, the hospital's community, and the potential fund-raising contributors of the hospital. This public, external market is not as clearly defined and is a much more difficult challenge for public relations directors and hospital management.

Most hospitals are involved in publishing public relations material and literature for their constituents. Hospitals commonly publish booklets containing patient or employee information. Frequently they publish their own internal newspapers, institutional brochures, or even annual reports for the internal group. The hospital administrator and management team initiate most of these internal publications. The hospital's patient audience has the greatest need for this type of published material and information, but unfortunately for the hospital, there is only a brief period in which to get its message across to most of its patients.

Some hospitals televise videos, and nearly every hospital has a Web site that builds an important image (and can be an important recruiting tool). Written publications are still important and may include the following:

- *A patient information booklet*—This booklet contains information that familiarizes the patient with the hospital's environment, gives the dos and don'ts of being a patient, and focuses on visitor information. This booklet should strive to be a warm communiqué, and it is an excellent opportunity to promote a positive image.

- *An employee information handbook*—This gives the employee the rules of employment, lists the employee's rights and obligations, and frequently outlines in some detail the fringe benefits available as an employee. This is a PR opportunity.

- *A hospital newsletter*—Typically, this is done by a local printer and is not generally of the quality of the mass media with which most of us are familiar. The newsletter may be published infrequently, perhaps once a month or once a quarter. The reporting staff is usually made up of amateur writers and reporters from within the hospital. However, it is a source of information, and if done properly, it is enjoyed by employee groups.

- *An institutional brochure*—This is available to internal groups, the board of trustees, and volunteers. It usually presents the history of the hospital, the philosophy of the institution, and the mission, vision, and core values of the hospital.

- *The annual report*—When a hospital publishes a formal annual report, it is usually done with quality printing and a high degree of expertise in its layout. The report is used for internal purposes of the medical staff, board of trustees, and employees, and it is frequently sent to other hospitals and to some external public constituents. Annual reports summarize the operational highlights of the year and usually list key management and medical staff.

Perhaps the most common relationship with the hospital's outside public is through mass media or press relations. The media provides a source for getting the hospital's message to the community. The hospital has specific objectives it wants to accomplish—mainly to keep its outside public informed, to improve or build a positive image for the hospital in the community, and to attempt to gain some influence on what the mass media report in the health care arena. The public relations department commonly uses press releases to keep in touch with the media and, accordingly, the public.

When a hospital embarks upon a capital fundraising campaign or annual fundraising effort, it must solicit its public, usually in written form. Though hospitals might not consider this a function of public relations, it clearly is since many letters of solicitation are sent out. Often, costly folders or brochures are developed and sent, usually through direct mail, to gain a specific reaction, namely, to raise funds from the hospital's external public.

Hospital Advertising

Advertising can be utilized to build the hospital's image or to sell a particular product. For example, a hospital may purchase billboards depicting a picture of the hospital with the tag line "Ready when you need us." This is clearly an *image* ad. As an alternative, the hospital may sell a particular *product* such as its ED depicted on the same type of billboard, with the tag line, "Seen in 30 minutes or your visit is free." This clearly touts the speed and efficiency of the ED crew. Both types of ads have their appropriate places.

Hospitals are getting involved increasingly in advertising. Today, more than half of hospitals' marketing budgets are spent on advertising. In fact, advertising has a major role to play in the entire marketing process, in both not-for-profit and profit-making activities in this country. Hospital advertising is a great way to promote facts related to hospital services and space facilities.

Hospitals are finding that they can have advertising tailored to their professional needs and can select very specific *target markets*. For example, they can target their advertising efforts toward physicians who may be interested in utilizing the hospital. Frequently, hospitals think about advertising as a way to increase activity in less frequently used services of the hospital. For example, prospective obstetrical patients may be attracted by a family-centered maternity room that has been advertised in the local newspaper, on television, or on the Web.

In general, hospital advertising 1) informs the public, 2) persuades the public, and 3) reminds the public. Mass production has created an economy of abundance. In this context, hospitals are competitive institutions. The federal government reports that there are too many hospital beds in this country. Because of this, it is logical to conclude that hospitals will turn to lessons learned by the for-profit retailing industry—that people can be persuaded to use one service in place of another. The hospital can make its product or service known and sell its benefits and features. It can employ advertising to remind the utilizing public to continue to use the service. It can remind them of the reasons they were satisfied with the hospital and what brought them there in the first place.

There are many reasons for hospitals to spend money on advertising. For one, the hospital's patients may need information on how to prevent disease and illness. They may need guidance on good nutrition or on how a woman can self-administer breast examinations. Another reason is that hospital patients need to understand the health care system and understand how preventive medicine programs interact with health care professionals. For example, patients might want to know where cancer screening is available and where children can receive immunizations. Advertising helps to inform hospital patients how to properly access the basics in the health care system. The hospital can also advertise to remind patients of services such as the newly remodeled ED, the new birthing center, or expanded clinic hours. Hospital advertising can convey this type of information to improve the image not only of the advertising hospital but the entire hospital industry's image as well. Hospitals are likely to be interested in advertising along these lines since such efforts are closely related to their mission of health education.

SALES

As hospitals become more businesslike and competitive, the sales function is growing in popularity. Some hospitals now have a dedicated sales force that reports directly to marketing executives or others in top management. These sales forces have proven to be effective, especially regarding certain restrictive services/products like occupational health, smoking cessation, sports medicine, or weight loss. Hospitals also use telemarketing and, of course, the invaluable hospital Internet Web site as sales tools.

This same sales force can be effective for physician recruiting and for educating doctors who are not on staff on the wonderful array of services the hospital offers.

BRANDING

Many hospitals are engaged in "branding," which identifies everything they do as originating from the same entity. To help understand branding, look at the example from Japan in the industrial giant Honda. After successfully manufacturing and marketing motorcycles, Honda introduced automobiles and then generators, chain saws, and countless other motorized products, all bearing the brand "Honda." In like manner, large hospitals with good reputations open clinics, long-term care facilities, home health agencies, durable medical equipment stores, etc., all with their hospital name as an attempt to brand the product as that of the same quality as the hospital.

MARKET RESEARCH

Market research is one of the most critical duties of the marketing department—one that hospitals make assumptions about or often overlook. The value of market research is that it provides information pertaining to the wants and needs of the hospital's patients, provides information about the local demographics, informs management of what the competition is doing, and provides information about physicians the hospital may want to recruit. Specifically, it can generate information concerning perceptions, preferences, and potential demand. Hospitals use various market research techniques. These include demographic analysis, direct mail and telephone surveys, personal interviews, and focus groups. Focus groups are usually volunteers of interest to the client that are paid to be interviewed in depth with open-ended questions about a single particular issue, for example, "Why did you choose to use Hospital A when you delivered your first baby?"

MARKET STUDIES AND MARKET AUDITS

Hospitals must become familiar with certain key concepts in the marketing process if they are to be successful. Perhaps the best place to begin is with a marketing study. A market study is simply a systematic, objective, critical way of appraising a market in which the hospital is interested. The marketing program can then be fine tuned toward the target in question. There are several steps in this study, which are:

1. Identify the kinds of information to be gathered in order to evaluate market or patient relations.
2. Set about collecting this data and information.
3. Evaluate the data and information that was collected.
4. Evaluate the amount of resources and effort needed to have a significant presence in that market.

As in an accounting audit, a market audit is an examination of how a process is being undertaken—in particular to marketing, the use of resources. Where are we spending our resources, and are they still being correctly allocated in the best manner? Do we have the necessary Web sites in place? Are we allocating too much to television? Are we overlooking drive-time and radio? Are there key billboards that we should purchase? What have our surveys shown about our effectiveness? Has our share of the market increased as a result of our expenditures?

Because many think that the physician is the principle target of a hospital's marketing program (after all, the hospital sits empty until a physician admits a patient), a common marketing audit in use by hospitals is the physician audit. This informs hospital management of how many physicians are admitting patients, the type of patients by payor category per physician compared to the same physician a year ago, how many surgeons are operating, etc. This will set a base line by which to measure progress. Other marketing audits include dollars spent compared to procedures, admissions, and surgeries performed.

After a marketing audit has been completed, it may become clear to the hospital that it has more than one kind of audience or public. The various audiences with which the hospital works are called segments or market segments. A market segment is a distinct group of patients or potential patients that can be separated from another group. For example, it is common to divide patients by type of insurance—Medicare, Medicaid, Blue Cross, etc. It is also common to divide patients by age or by required service, e.g., OB, pediatrics, cardiac, etc. Frequently, patients are divided by income level or geographic location. The different ways of categorizing the hospital's patients identify particular market segments.

After completing an audit and identifying a hospital's different segments, it is important for the hospital to realize that the patients and competing hospitals have an image of the hospital. Where the hospital fits into this image spectrum is called the hospital's *positioning strategy*.

It is important to understand the concept of positioning when trying to determine what programs the hospital should invest in and sponsor. To use an illustration from commercial business, the Avis position was not clear until the company finally adopted the slogan that they were number two. This move had great success because Avis did not position itself directly opposite its number one competitor, but in fact differentiated itself from its competition. Put into hospital language, if a neighboring hospital has a superior cardiology unit, perhaps the hospital with the lesser cardiology unit should promote its outpatient pediatrics services. It would position itself as different from its competition, become successful and strong, while carving out its own unique niche.

With the concept of a marketing niche, segment, or positioning in mind, the marketing program can proceed with the classic four Ps of marketing. The objective is to put the right *product* (in the hospital's position, this is a service) into the right *place* (proper location) at the right *price* with the proper *promotion*.

With regard to the right product, it should be remembered that hospitals do not really sell products; they sell services. They sell the benefit or satisfaction a patient may get from receiving services. This is the hospital's product. Ideally, a hospital should conduct inventories or marketing audits frequently to determine what its product and benefits should be. Hospitals should regularly analyze their service programs.

A good example regarding place, or location, of health care can be seen in satellite outpatient clinics or in medical office buildings that are placed near a hospital. Such hospitals have placed their services in the right location. They are convenient and responsive to the patient.

Now that the federal government and other large insurers reimburse hospitals for care, price, the third P, may have become less important to the hospital industry than to retail business. There is still, however, a mentality of price, especially in the small portion of the market that purchases services directly—for example, elective surgery not covered by insurance. The market is somewhat sensitive to the cost for an hour in the operating room, a 4-day stay in the nursery, or a standard urinalysis charge. Cost still must be considered in the total marketing program and especially when negotiating with HMOs.

The last P, promotion, refers to the classic marketing activities that hospitals have undertaken. It also refers to advertising and to innovative ways of promoting products (for example, premiums and incentives that could be offered to certain people). Hospitals must be sensitive to the ethical issue of promotion of health services.

It is important for hospitals to understand in detail the strategies and tactics of the marketing process. If they want to attract new physicians, to develop effective programs, to retain qualified personnel, and to remain current in their delivery services, marketing can be a great asset.

FUND-RAISING

Most not-for-profit hospitals rely on donations and fund-raising efforts as a source of needed funds. Fund-raising may be divided into two general categories: 1) annual giving programs and 2) capital or special purpose campaigns. A hospital's regular annual giving programs are usually conducted by the hospital's development staff. Hospitals often have a section or part of their organization devoted to fund-raising. This section or department is referred to as the development office. Hospitals frequently use outside consultants to assist them on special or capital campaigns. Many of the tactics used to solicit funds draw on proven marketing methods, including direct mail, a special section of the hospital's Web site, direct contacts, solicitation of individuals, and special events. Major sources targeted for giving include wealthy individuals, large business corporations, and foundations.

CHAPTER REVIEW

1. What is marketing? How is it different from public relations?
2. What are the four Ps of marketing?
3. What is a target market?
4. What are focus groups?
5. Give five examples of written publications important to the hospital's marketing effort.
6. How is image advertising different from product line advertising?
7. What is branding?
8. Give four examples of a hospital's market research effort.
9. What is a physician audit?
10. Describe positioning and tell why it is important.
11. What are two methods of hospital fundraising?
12. Contact the marketing director of a large hospital in your city and discuss the market channel. What has their hospital done "upstream" to build an intake program to acquire patients (for example, free standing clinics) and what has been done "downstream" for continued care (for example, home health, a retail outlet for durable medical equipment, a long-term care facility)?

Chapter 26

Planning

INTRODUCTION

Planning is a roadmap. It is a careful analysis, based on facts and evidence, of where and what the organization is, how it relates to its environment and competition, where it wants to go or to become, how quickly the developments will happen, and who is responsible for each segment in the process. To quote the famous baseball player Yogi Berra, "If you don't know where you are going, you could end up somewhere else." Planning makes management sense and common sense as well, particularly now that third parties and regulatory agencies are all pushing the hospital into a more competitive environment. Administrators see the changing demands of the population. The needs of physicians are increasing. The matter of solvency and appropriate reimbursement mandates budgetary planning. Today the hospital's survival is truly contingent upon its ability to make the correct strategic decisions for its future course of action.

THE EVOLUTION OF PLANNING

In the early 1950s, about 10 hospital councils, located mostly in large urban cities, had made some progress on capital planning in their respective regions. After 1955, more and more agencies were specifically structured to aid in community planning, and definite planning programs were set up for metropolitan hospital areas.

Planning continued to evolve through the 1950s and 1960s. Planning was generally synonymous with developing new facilities in a rapidly expanding health care market. There was a major concentration on the development, construction, and design of a hospital's physical plant. The focus in the 1970s was characterized by the development or expansion of programs, services, and products. In the 1980s, planning moved beyond the institution to the external environment with an emphasis in developing outside relationships. Today, partly because of the oversupply of beds in many areas and the tightening of government regulations, planning may mean a great deal more than expansion and growth; planning is used to ensure that a hospital's services are necessary, appropriate, and profitable and that those services will thrive in the future. Recently it has become common for hospitals to develop associations, shared services, or linkages with other health providers as part of their planning process.

Hospitals are looking seriously at vertical and horizontal growth in the industry. For example, they are exploring home care, primary care, and other forms of subacute care that relate directly to the hospital (horizontal integration); they are looking additionally to clinics and long term care that could be *sources* of patients and places to *send* patients (vertical integration). Many hospitals are joining in not-for-profit multisystems of one kind or another.

THE HOSPITAL'S LONG-RANGE PLAN

It is to the advantage of a hospital to do sound, practical planning for the future—particularly now that there are so many competitive forces, e.g., freestanding surgery centers owned by physicians and new governmental regulations impacting the hospital's environment. The changing patterns of medical practice include the shift from acute inpatients to ambulatory medicine, the mushrooming of biomedical technology with its impact on the hospital's operation costs and future, and shifts in demographics and community needs. These changing patterns are especially important in urban areas where age, insurance coverage, and mobility are constant factors in hospital planning. Finally, changing economic conditions—particularly in the availability of money to carry out the hospital's plans—and increased legislation and regulations will affect the hospital. These factors must all be placed into the planning combination in order to derive a list of options that will serve the hospital in the future.

WHO SHOULD DO THE HOSPITAL'S PLANNING?

The hospital's planning effort is usually led or initiated by the CEO but generally involves active participation from the senior management team, the board, and the medical staff. The CEO may also receive assistance from the hospital's own planning department, if they have one, or from outside consultants.

As the person who is primarily responsible for carrying out the board's decisions, the administrator or CEO participates actively in planning deliberations. Usually the CEO determines the planning process and suggests to the board the various options available in making long-range planning decisions.

The medical staff's role is also critical. The medical staff must identify changes in the health care needs of the community and suggest new options on how the hospital could meet these changing medical needs. They are also the ones who will be using any new technology that the hospital purchases. Medical staff members are spokespersons for advancing technology and can advise the board's planning committee on how this technology will influence the hospital's plan. Another byproduct of having the medical staff participate in planning is that staff members can become acquainted with the problems facing hospital management in planning for the future, usually in an environment of limited resources.

The Strategic Planning Process

Hospitals generally engage in sequential planning in order to create their strategic plan (also sometimes known as a "5 Year Plan"). An environmental scan is done as a first step in order to analyze the political, competitive, regulatory, social, economic, and technological environment. Following that is an assessment of both the internal and external environments of the hospital's needs. This evaluation step is commonly referred to as a SWOT analysis; it evaluates the institution's strengths, weaknesses, opportunities, and threats. Strengths and weaknesses are a form of internal analysis; opportunities and threats allow the hospital to examine the external environment. An essential element is to examine the demographic trends of the area to note potential pitfalls.

Once the hospital's internal and external environments have been analyzed, the hospital decides what it wants to do and be in a broad sense. This decision involves reviewing the hospital's mission statement to insure that it is current. The mission statement is what the hospital is all about, or what it stands for. The mission statement expresses the hospital's philosophy and details what community services, research, educational commitments, and major offerings the hospital will provide. Mission statements should be simple and even short enough to be incorporated on an employee's name badge. An example might be "Delivering excellent care, benchmarked to international standards." Mission statements are usually written through a joint effort of the CEO and Board of Directors.

A vision statement is a statement of hope. It is where the hospital wants to be in the future, or where it sees itself in 10–15 years. Usually the CEO writes the vision statement.

The hospital then develops goals and objectives for accomplishing its mission. Alternatives for accomplishing goals are evaluated. Goals, strategies, and tactics for achieving those goals are made part of the plan with a measurable timetable included. A careful market analysis is usually undertaken to correctly understand the competition and competitive factors, and then timetables are agreed upon for the above-mentioned goals and who is responsible for attaining the goals. After the plan is approved and implemented, it must be evaluated and refined on a regular basis, usually yearly or biyearly. In summary, strategic planning involves 1) an environmental scan, 2) examining and assessing the organization's strengths, weaknesses, opportunities, and threats (SWOT), 3) writing a mission and vision statement (and communicating it to all employees and the public), 4) setting goals and objectives, then 5) assigning a timetable and 6) who is responsible for each goal that was set. As mentioned before, a periodic review of the process is necessary to assess if the hospital is on track or new goals should be set.

LEVELS OF LONG-RANGE PLANNING

A hospital's plan may well have different levels of involvement. These could be 1) the CEO and the board creating the strategic plan, 2) the senior level division executives (DON, CFO, COO, etc.) then creating the tactical plan, and finally, 3) the department directors fleshing out the operations.

BENEFITS OF PLANNING

Proper long-range planning will improve the hospital's overall ability to deal with the future. Specifically, it will show the following benefits:

- It will establish a systematic basis for relating to the allocation of specific and frequently limited resources in the hospital's future.
- It will ensure that the hospital continues to look at its mission statement and its resources to carry out its mission.
- It will continue to test the viability of the hospital by integrating budgets with long-range strategic plans.
- It will give management more control because it will have a better idea of where it is going; this will also guide management's day-to-day operations.
- It will give the hospital a standard for management against which it can evaluate and measure performance.

PLANNING NEW FACILITIES

Facility planning involves defining the hospital's facility needs over the next several years. The facilities should not drive the plan, but rather form should follow function. A master site and facilities plan needs to be agreed upon and followed if the hospital's planning is going to be efficient.

Planners today have a big advantage in that they can very easily access vital data on the Web using a host of search engines. For example, if the hospital wishes to expand the neonatal intensive care unit, there are existing formulas that predict the number of beds needed for any given time period, based on the number of births and the number of current neonatal intensive care unit (NICU) patients and the anticipated population growth.

One other issue a health care facility planner must be aware of is a certificate of need (CON). Many states have become involved in limiting care due to areas of the state being overbedded. In such cases, health care entities must apply for a certificate of need, which demonstrates that the proposed service is lacking or insufficient. This will limit the number of facilities built. Other states, such as Texas, have abolished the CON process, reasoning that economic forces should be allowed to work.

CHAPTER REVIEW

1. What is a plan? Why plan?
2. What is a mission statement? A vision statement?
3. Why must upper management be involved in planning? Why can't it just retain a consultant service?

DISCUSSION QUESTIONS

1. Should the hospital involve local leaders in the planning process? Why or why not?
2. Does the CON process save taxpayers money or does it spend taxpayer money on unnecessary agencies and attorney fees?
3. How often should a hospital undertake planning?
4. Should a hospital periodically change its mission? Why or why not?
5. Discuss why planning is very important, but is wasteful without "implementation" and then "execution" (of the plan).

Part X

The US and World Health Care Systems

Chapter 27

The US Medical Care System

INTRODUCTION

We commonly define a system as a related or connected arrangement of things that forms a single entity; a set. Therefore, a health care system is a set of mechanisms through which human resources, facilities, and medical technology are organized by means of administrative structures. The system offers integrated services in sufficient quantity and quality to meet most of the population's demand. However, in referring to the US health care system's structure, its critics have sometimes called it a nonsystem. This observation reflects pluralism within the hospital structure rather than a lack of system. The American system has not been the product of a grand central design, but rather has evolved over the past 250 years into a "patchwork quilt."

Many think that the American medical system offers at least three classes of care: middle-class care; second-class care; and the narrow and limited "princely" care given to the elite and superwealthy. Because our society has much more knowledge than know-how, there has been progress in medical science but a failure to make it accessible in equal proportions to all segments of our society.

The type of medical care a person receives depends upon where the person lives and how much money the person has. Better care is given to those living near university medical centers or the sophisticated urban teaching hospitals. A fact of American life is that medicine is usually a middle-class institution, with some elite care for the rich, and some subpar care for those without insurance.

Of course, physicians serve the poor and practice in underprivileged areas, but have they really been trained to concentrate on taking care of the largest segment, the middle class? In this chapter we will describe but not defend the medical care system (or the sickness system) that exists in the United States today. Four *medical institutional elements* that are related are 1) the outreach element, 2) the outpatient element, 3) the inpatient element, and 4) the extended element; and one additional element that affects the institutional components: the community element. These different components or elements of the system will be examined.

THE SYSTEM'S GOALS

Before examining each of the components in detail, it is important to learn the general goals of our nation's health care system. These goals are presently being met in varying degrees based on geographic locale and economic status. Some of the gaps in the medical care system are seen when the goals are weighed against what is actually happening in the medical care world. Traditional US medical systems have generally aimed at the following goals:

- Health care should be available to all people.
- Health care should be both psychologically and socially acceptable to all those using it.
- Health care should be delivered with reasonable quality.
- Health care should be comprehensive but should stress maximum economic efficiency.

In short, the major issues facing a health care system are access to care, quality of care, and cost of care.

While these goals are noble, they still need to be weighed against some fundamental questions such as the following:[a]

- What place and importance should be given to health care in managing our political and social systems?
- What kind of quality life should we expect from our medical care?

---

[a]Notice how these goals are similar to the social justice issues discussed in Chapter 23.

- How much and what kind of health does a society need in order to be a good society?
- Who is to provide this health care, pay for it, and take responsibility for it?

Given these goals and questions, let us examine the various components of the medical care system.

OUTREACH ELEMENT

The first component of the medical care system is the outreach element. In essence, the traditional system attempts to meet the patient's primary medical care needs through outreach programs. These programs are generally decentralized. They are scattered activities. Outreach activities may include private physicians' offices in the community, health care centers, group practices, ambulatory care arrangements, and outpatient activities of providers such as health maintenance organizations (HMOs).

Traditionally, most patients in the United States have received care through their primary care physician (or the solo practitioner). This is the most common example of the system's outreach component. Private or solo practitioners provide the bulk of the US outreach activity. At the same time, the urban poor may use city health clinics, public health nurses, or visiting nurses associations. The outreach element also includes groups like school nurses, sophisticated group practices that are freestanding from hospitals, the myriad of storefront clinic arrangements that are found in urban centers, and the multispecialty offices that deliver Medicaid services and proliferate in some of our urban areas. Other social agencies have been involved in outreach from time to time. Churches often are involved in screening activities and in providing centers for referral through physicians or hospitals. This outreach phase is the beginning of the referral sequence for many patients in our present medical care system.

In outreach, we are able to distinguish two classes of care. As we have noted, one type of care is offered to middle-class consumers, and the other is given to the poor. These two groups take different routes to care, with the middle class historically being served by the private practitioner and the primary care physician, and the poor served by emergency departments or city health clinics.

There is a maldistribution of physicians; urban areas and large parts of the inner city, as well as our depressed rural areas, often lack physicians. Rarely does one find members of the middle class using city health clinics, neighborhood health centers, or mental health program clinics. It is much more common for the medically indigent (those who cannot afford medical insurance—either the unemployed or those working for an employer who is too small to afford coverage for the employees) to use these sites. The real and significant difference between the two populations is how the middle class and the poor class are referred into the medical institutions in the system. Clearly, the two groups are not referred with the same social and psychological acceptance.

The outreach component of our traditional system is probably in trouble. An increasing problem is that the middle class is also having difficulty being referred into the other sectors of the medical care system. Witness the growth in physician referral programs used by numerous hospitals as a service and marketing technique. Even some middle-class patients may now have some difficulty finding primary care practitioners in quiet suburban areas. A troubling fact is that many middle-class consumers may not be able to guide themselves through the medical care system. The patients want physicians to take care of the whole person, not just the orthopedic, urologic, or psychiatric problem. This new problem for the middle class is the same one that the poor have experienced for years—lack of conveniences and accessibility to quality care. For citizens in managed care plans, this may not be the same problem.

OUTPATIENT ELEMENT

The second component of our health system is the outpatient component. This system part embodies traditional hospital clinics and outpatient services. Historically, clinics located in large urban areas were created for teaching purposes or for serving the poor. Today the outpatient elements also probably mean the hospital emergency departments.

With the passage of the Emergency Medical Treatment and Active Labor Act (EMTALA) in 1986, Medicare participating hospitals must stabilize patients before transferring them to other institutions, thereby preventing "patient dumping." In effect, this means that a hospital participating in the Medicare program (nearly 100% of all hospitals) must see every patient who presents to the emergency department, regardless of the patients' ability to pay. Patients who do not have a family physician or cannot afford one often utilize the emergency department as their primary care physician.

Studies have shown that more than 60 percent of all emergency cases that visit emergency departments are probably not true clinical emergencies. This is further evidence of the problem of access in our medical care system.

What are other reasons why so many patients use the emergency department? If we trace the evolution of the emergency department, we see that the volume began to increase sharply after World War II, and it has continued to grow steadily since that time. The emergency departments remain the one marketplace of medical care where there is an interface between the middle class and the poor. Both groups accept this service. There is no stigma in going to an emergency department. Nevertheless, there is definitely a stigma attached to waiting on a hard wooden bench in a teaching clinic in one of our large urban medical centers. These clinics are the embodiment of the two-class system, but change and improvement are taking place. Many large teaching hospitals in urban centers find themselves serving a disproportionate number of poor and older citizens. In spite of the need to train physicians in their clinics, serious questions are being raised about the future of university teaching clinics due to the drain of resources to the hospital. Many of these teaching clinics have reorganized into group practices.

There have been traditionally few financial barriers in going to the emergency department. It is open for emergencies, urgent care, and other routine services, and it is not primarily interested in a patient's ability to pay. It is common to see an executive sitting next to a welfare recipient in a busy city emergency department. This is the one place in the outpatient component that has bandaged the gap in the health care delivery system.

Ambulance services are an outpatient activity that has taken on increased status with the advent of paramedics, cardiopulmonary resuscitation teams, and electronic monitoring. However, for millions who live in cities, there are still two kinds of ambulance services. One is the municipal service, which is really an extension of the police ambulance or fire department. The other is the community ambulance staffed primarily for the people who can afford ambulances. This is another example of a multitiered system.

INPATIENT ELEMENT

The third element is the inpatient (hospital) component. This is represented and characterized by the hospital bed. Over the last decade, there has been a significant change in the classification of beds. The number of general medical/surgical beds has decreased as the number of intensive care beds has increased. Hospitals continue to use the bed as the benchmark of occupancy, service, and financing, yet only 10 percent of the health needs of patients in our system are cared for in the inpatient part of the hospital.

The difficulties that are inherent in the hospital system stem from dependency on the hospital bed. For example, one model of the economy of hospitals indicates that hospitals are controlled by their medical staff who seek to maximize their own income, and in so doing, they use the hospital bed extensively, which begins the vicious circle of increased hospital cost. As it now stands, the economics of the hospital requires that the beds be filled for the hospital to stay solvent. The present inpatient system has a great deal of overlapping coverage or duplication of services. This is why mergers, shared services, and linkages are now in vogue and will undoubtedly increase and become more common. This trend may be a single step toward improving care as well as toward holding a line on costs. Still, hospitals will need to strive for productivity, quality, and better bottom lines through efficiency.

An interesting fact in the inpatient system is that physicians are regarded by hospitals as both consumers and providers. Hospitals provide facilities not for the patient but for the physicians who admit the patients. In turn, physicians provide care to their patients and are therefore themselves providers. Understanding this arrangement is critical in identifying the control valve in the cost of medical care.

EXTENDED ELEMENT

The fourth element in the system is the extended component. Included in this area are such things as long-term care hospitals, home care programs, skilled nursing facilities (SNFs) (facilities that provide less than acute care as those found in a hospital, and more care than a long-term care facility), durable medical equipment companies, visiting nurses, hospice care, wellness programs, freestanding oncology centers, birthing centers, independent laboratories, rehabilitation centers, and certain other specialty hospitals.

The scientific professional component that has done such a magnificent job in our inpatient facilities seems to be lagging in the treatment provided in our long-term care programs. The extended component seems to receive relatively little support and therefore may deteriorate and become the weakest link in the system. For an illustration, one has only to look at the deplorable conditions of some of our nation's long-term care facilities.

Community Element

The fifth and final element is noninstitutional. This is the community component. The community can be viewed from multiple perspectives. The first is a view of the community as a consumer group, those who use health care facilities. Today, consumers are better educated than ever about health care and are an active group.

The community element also includes health work force resources, that is, the medical training programs in our medical schools and in our teaching hospitals. Aligned to this work force element are labor unions. They can be a force in the supply and demand function for labor in some parts of the nation. Another element is demographic shifts. The aging of US citizens, as well as diseases like AIDS, will also affect our hospitals' long-range plans.

Finally, there is the role of the federal and state governments as part of the community component. In this context, we must consider dollars that are spent on health care through the federal government. Americans spend billions on health care yearly, with much of this expenditure through Medicare and Medicaid programs.

Apart from these aspects, the community element also includes private insurance plans and health maintenance organizations, as well as other types of managed health care programs. Also included in the community element are lifestyle changes and the rapid rise in medical technology. Beyond this are educational, community, and environmental health components such as pollution control. Finally, we must include the politics of health care in the community component.

The US medical care system can be viewed as having numerous strengths (technology, modern facilities, solid training programs, etc.) but also numerous weaknesses (lack of an overall structure leading to wasteful duplication of services, questionable access to care, need for quality improvements, etc.).

There is a need for reform to change this "patchwork quilt" system in order to provide uniform access to care, decreased expenditures, and improved quality. That is a challenge for all of us.

CHAPTER REVIEW

1. Why is the US health care system called a "patchwork quilt?"
2. What are three major issues that must be addressed by a health care system?
3. What are four medical institutional elements and a fifth affecting element?
4. Discuss ways of changing the misdistribution of physicians in the US. What incentives or disincentives can be undertaken to persuade new physicians to move to rural areas?
5. What are the three classes of care discussed in the chapter? How can care be made more equitable?
6. Discuss the pros and cons of universal health care. Examine the Canadian system and compare it to what you understand is provided in the US. Why is the topic of universal healthcare destined to be one of the leading political issues in the very near future? Why is industry suddenly supporting such an effort toward universal coverage?

Chapter 28

The US Health Care System Compared to the World

<table>
<tr><td colspan="2" align="center">**Key Terms**</td></tr>
<tr><td>Access to care</td><td>Quality of care</td></tr>
<tr><td>Cost of care</td><td></td></tr>
</table>

INTRODUCTION

The reader has developed an understanding of key elements of the health care system and hospitals as they are managed in the United States. What about the rest of the world? What similarities are present? What differences should be noted?

THE UNITED STATES

It may surprise readers to learn that the United States has the most expensive system in the world, costing 14 percent of the gross domestic product, yet it does not have the highest life expectancy or the lowest infant mortality rate; the United States is ranked 37th among countries in overall performance by the World Health Organization.[1,2]

In comparing health care systems, it is a good idea to use commonalities so that apples are compared to apples and oranges are compared to oranges. Three important items that can be used to compare all health care systems are 1) the cost of care, 2) access to care, and 3) quality of care.

COST OF CARE AND ACCESS TO CARE

As has been noted, the cost of care in the United States is the highest in the world, with spending at 15 percent of GDP. All other countries, except the very poor ones, are more likely to spend approximately 9 percent of GDP. This becomes more remarkable when we learn that nearly all countries give health care to nearly 100 percent of their citizens, yet in the United States, there are usually about 44,000,000 (some estimate about 15 percent of the population) without health care insurance coverage.[3] We can then say that nearly all other countries have access to care at about 100 percent; the United States has access to care at about 85 percent.

Chapter 27 explained how the evolution of the US health care system resulted in a figurative patchwork quilt. Not only is the system itself a patchwork quilt, but the system of health care payment in the United States is as well . . . some citizens have Medicare, some Medicaid, some have third-party payer coverage, some have governmental coverage such as the Veterans Administration or the Indian Health Service, and others have no coverage at all. The last group often is dependent on the emergency departments of hospitals, very often waiting until it is too late for care. The movement for universal access has never succeeded in the United States, although it has been attempted under seven US presidents.

If care does cost more in the United States, why does it cost more? Some reasons that add up to higher health care costs in the United States are: 1) the United States tends to spend more on technology with every hospital vying to get the latest and greatest machines so as to attract the most admitting physicians; 2) US physicians, on average, are the best paid in the world; 3) many US physicians practice defensive medicine to avoid lawsuits; and 4) there are fraud and abuse issues of health care providers billing the government for procedures that were not done.

QUALITY OF CARE

Whether the United States ranks high in quality issues seems to depend on what statistics are reviewed. For example, the US infant mortality rate, as measured in 2003 by the Organization for Economic Development and Cooperation, was 6.9 deaths per 1,000 live births–this is twice the rate of that in Japan with 3.2 deaths, and 20 to 50 percent higher than Canada, France, Germany, and the United Kingdom.

On the other hand, another measure of quality is the effectiveness of disease treatment. According to a World Health Organization study in 2001, the United States has the lowest mortality rate for breast, prostate, and colon/rectal cancer when compared to the countries of Canada, France, Germany, and the United

Kingdom. However, many would argue that mortality rates are not a good measure of the effectiveness of a country in treating many varying diseases.

OVERSEAS OPPORTUNITIES

The world is shrinking and it is now common for executives to find opportunities all over the world. During this writer's relatively short time in health care administration (1985–2005), there have been offers to manage a hospital in Nigeria, transition a clinic into a hospital in Moscow, open a hospital in Malaysia, and offer advice to a 342-bed acute-care facility in Saudi Arabia, which is my current position.

The hospital where I'm working in Saudi Arabia births about 250 babies per month. It also cares for about 10,000 patients a month in the emergency department, performs nearly every type of surgery except transplants and heart surgery, and operates a multitude of clinics and dental facilities. The hospital has recently applied for JCI accreditation.

Students should find similar opportunities as they build their careers. For example, they could start in Los Angeles, transfer to Dubai for a few years, and then manage a facility in Calcutta. Administrators will find hospitals much the same the world over, using similar technology, hiring physicians with similar skills, and competing for a nursing staff that is even more mobile.

CHAPTER REVIEW

1. What are the three key areas usually used to compare health care systems?
2. Why is health care in the United States more expensive than in the rest of the world?
3. What portion of the US population does not have health insurance?
4. Where does the United States rank in the world regarding health care according to the WHO?
5. What are the criteria used by the WHO to rank the quality of health and health care in countries? What nations rank in the top 10 and why?
6. If you were to obtain a healthcare executive position outside of the United States, what obstacles would you expect to find during your first 3 months and during your first year in the foreign nation?

NOTES

1. World Health Organization, 2000, http://www.who.int.
2. US Census Bureau, 1999.
3. US Census Bureau, 2000.

Appendix A

Case Studies

This appendix contains 10 case studies, which should challenge you in your quest to understand the modern medical center and its environment. All of the cases are presented from the perspective of the reader as the hospital's CEO. Some of the cases present bioethical dilemmas; others may include challenges relating to marketing, planning, management, legal issues, the medical staff, or other issues.

The cases are designed to illustrate problems that can arise in management, both common problems and unusual problems, and then to provoke group discussion with the team assigned the case. This should simulate how the CEO and management team would engage the issue within their hospital. Not all of the cases can be solved from the text material alone. The author suggests that this illustrates the real world; executives often face problems for which they have no experience, training, or precedence. Students are certainly invited to use other resources.

The external environment of the hospital is changed with each case, some are set in cities, others in rural areas, yet others are not described because of the irrelevance to the case.

The cases are:

1. Towel? What Towel?
2. Water; Water Everywhere (3 parts)
3. Problems for the New Administrator (3 parts)
4. I'm Calling the EEOC and Filing a Complaint
5. Controls and Indicators for the Ship

6. The Case of Jill
7. The Need to Communicate
8. Adding a New Service to the Hospital
9. The Case of "Baby B"
10. The Case of the Relocated Management Team

Case 1:

Towel? What Towel?

You arrive at your office and find Dr. Ratliff waiting to see you. Dr. Ratliff is an experienced pathologist; one of the best physicians in the hospital. When he looks worried, you understand it is time to worry.

He begins with, "Chief, I was in my office this morning when surgery sent what appeared to be a large hairy softball. I bisected it and found a large green towel with the hospital's name on it." How could this have happened? Stunned, you ask the physician to continue.

Dr. Ratliff continued. "Well, you know the tax assessor's wife, Mrs. Bradley? She had a hysterectomy about three months ago; Dr. Estelle did the surgery. Apparently, he has a technique that uses a hospital towel . . . after he opens the patient, he takes the hospital towel, which is folded and rolled up like a hot dog, and one of the surgery technicians uses the towel to retract the patient's tissue while the operation is conducted. Since Mrs. Bradley is overweight, some of her tissue covered the towel that no one noticed, and Dr. Estelle closed her up."

You think for a moment and ask, "Why didn't the nurses do a towel count at the completion of the surgery?"

Dr. Ratliff replies, "I thought the same thing and asked that of the surgery director. He told me, 'Hey, we count sponges, clamps, and other instruments, but we don't count towels. How can anyone leave an 18 x 24" green surgery towel in a patient? From now on, however, you had better believe that we'll count every towel.'"

"How did the patient discover that the towel might be inside her?" you ask.

Dr. Ratliff continues, "It seems that the patient began to notice a protruding lump, and the lump kept getting bigger. She went to a different doctor since Dr. Estelle and she had a falling out regarding her bill. This time she went to Dr. Gibson. Dr. Gibson palpated the area, x rayed it, then opened her up and found the towel. He says that he has not yet spoken with her; she is still in recovery."

DISCUSSION

What action do you deem to be appropriate? Whom should you contact? Does the patient have an action that meets the four necessary elements of negligence? Whom might her attorney name as defendants? How can you quickly act to mitigate possible damages?

Case 2:

Water; Water Everywhere

This case study is in three parts. You will derive the most value from the case if you stop reading when directed and discuss the points that have just occurred.

PART 1

As you left your office Friday afternoon, you were delighted that it had been raining for nearly a week. Your 177-bed hospital is located in an arid part of the state that sees a minimum amount of rain each year. The city's water supply comes from San Gabriel Creek, a spring-fed creek emanating from underground. In fact, this creek is the reason the Spaniards founded the city of San Gabriel nearly 400 years ago. The spring pumps 90 million gallons of water a day as the creek winds its way majestically through the center of the city of San Gabriel.

Sunday night at about 11:30, your phone rings. Rising from a deep sleep, you find it to be the vice president of nursing, Mr. Arthur. In your absence, Mr. Arthur is the acting CEO. While his voice is under control, you have never heard him sound so serious.

"Chief, do not try to come to the hospital; you won't make it. The entire town is flooded and the hospital is receiving casualties. When the sun comes up, predictions are that there will be hundreds of bodies floating all over town. San Gabriel Creek overflowed its banks and many houses have been torn from their foundations."

You agree that you probably cannot make it to the hospital, and you also feel that Mr. Arthur will need relief in his capacity as acting CEO when morning comes. You go back to bed and ponder what you have just heard.

Part 1 Discussion

Stop—please *do not* read further. What priorities will you set in the morning? After you've discussed this question, continue to Part 2.

PART 2

When morning comes, the floodwaters have receded and you are able to drive to the hospital. Upon arrival, you find approximately 80 very wet people sleeping in the hallways. You gather your team of the chief engineer, vice president of nursing, assistant administrator, and public relations director. You begin to receive damage reports from each.

The chief engineer reports that the hospital has not been directly affected by the flood due to its location near the top of a hill. He does reveal bad news, however; the city has lost its entire water supply, due to city water pumps being flooded. It is believed that the city's water supply could be out for as long as 30 days. The pumps were old and parts are no long available; the pumps will have to be replaced.

Mr. Arthur discloses that there were 12 people reported killed during the flood. More than 700 homes were swept away, but most people were able to evacuate swiftly. The hospital emergency department received 50 casualties during the night with nearly all being lacerations occurring from the flood.

When you ask Mr. Arthur about such surprisingly low casualties compared to the initial prediction, he reports, "The Red Cross arrived around 4 a.m. and set up emergency facilities at the civic center. There are about 500 people sleeping there. Our own staff, with the exception of about 10 to 12 people, was able to report to work this morning."

Ms. Nelson, the ancillary and support services director has some grim information. "There is no water supply to the hospital. We have lost our ability to do surgery because the air chillers are not working since they are water cooled. The surgery suite is no longer cool and the sterile packs are no longer sterile due to high humidity. Lacking the proper working facilities, patients cannot use their restrooms and dietary cannot prepare meals."

Part 2 Discussion

Stop—Please do not read further until you've discussed the following questions. What priorities do you set? What action do you take?

PART 3

That morning, you join a team of about 30 community leaders who have agreed to meet at the San Gabriel airport each morning. This team is comprised of key government officials, members of the sheriff's department, the state department of public safety, the police department, the border patrol, the Red Cross, the hospital, etc. The leadership of this organization has been ceded to the state department of public safety due to the resources they can provide and due to their experience in matters of this nature. The department's helicopter pilots have been looking for additional victims and have brought in search dogs. To date, 3 more bodies have been found, for a total of 15.

Regarding the water supply, it has been confirmed that the supply will be nonexistent for at least 30 days. Bottled water is being brought to the city and given to anyone who needs it. Many are driving outside of town to use showers provided by citizens with water wells.

The hospital has taken its surgical instruments to the local air force base, which has the ability to sterilize instruments in its dispensary. The hospital was able to obtain a water-pumping fire truck from the city and then connect it by a large hose to a water tanker truck from the air force base. The water truck was then connected to a city water pipe leading into the hospital and the fire truck began pumping water; the hospital gained its own water supply, replacing the water supply once furnished by the city. Every two hours, the water truck would leave to be replaced quickly by another water truck sitting directly behind it. In effect, your hospital has the only water supply in the entire city.

DISCUSSION

How do you think outside agencies evaluating the hospital would rate the hospital at each stage of the disaster? Why? What do you think the hospital should do to minimize likcly disasters in the future? What lessons have been learned from this?

Case 3:

Problems for the New Administrator

BACKGROUND

El Verde Memorial is a 98-bed acute-care hospital in a rural town of 35,000 citizens, located in Rojo County, a western US area of approximately 55,000 residents. The facility is the sole provider of medical care for the county, hosting an emergency department, the only ambulance service in the county, an OB department, pediatric services, three surgery suites, and other services normally expected.

The hospital is owned by the hospital district, an entity created by the state and partially supported by taxes. It is governed by a seven-person board of directors who are elected by the citizens of Rojo County for 2 year terms. The board hires the administrator, who serves at their will.

The citizens are proud of their hospital, which dates to 1954, having been constructed with Hill-Burton funds. The town is in the South and is in a very rural part of the state, located 150 miles from any larger cities, and it borders Mexico.

This rural municipality has 14 general practitioners (MDs and DOs), 3 general surgeons (2 who are in practice together), 2 cardiologists, 3 internal medicine specialists, 1 urologist, 3 OB/GYNs, and 2 pediatricians. All own their own buildings and practices. There are also 3 certified registered nurse anesthetists (CRNAs) who provide OR coverage for the surgeons.

The primary economic base for the county is sheep grazing; the sheep are shorn for wool and are shipped annually to market by rail. There are no feedlots; rather the county prides itself on organic farming and ranching, with many families contributing to the county's total output. There is a small military base, a US Border Patrol headquarters, a mall, and a recreation lake that attracts many tourists. The town's population grows dramatically in winter due to many Canadians and retirees from the Northern states fleeing south to escape colder climates. As the new hospital CEO, you are facing a major challenge during your first few months in office.

PART 1

The problem is that the hospital has no medical office building. This presents an obstacle in recruiting new physicians to move to El Verde. Where will you tell new physicians to locate their practices?

You submit a memorandum to the hospital's board of directors, proposing that a medical office building be constructed immediately next to the hospital, on property already owned, and that it be connected to the hospital by an overhead walkway.

You find that the medical staff initially is very surprised and then openly hostile to this proposed construction. They argue that their personal investments in their own offices will diminish with the hospital's construction and that they will be at a pronounced disadvantage with new physicians in a building next to the hospital.

Finally, the Chief of the Medical Staff says, "Are you aware of the economic might we physicians have? We are some of the biggest depositors in the El Verde Bank, and we can switch our money to Big Lake Bank. How do you think the two board members who work at El Verde Bank will feel about you when they learn our reason for switching banks? The Board can unappoint you just like they appointed you!"

Part 1 Discussion

Often an administrator faces issues where the medical staff acts against the financial interests of the hospital, such as building a free-standing outpatient surgical center or an imaging center in the immediate vicinity of the hospital. In this case study, the hospital is acting contrary to the best interests of some of the physicians by erecting a MOB to attract new physicians. Should a compromise be structured and, if so, what terms would you suggest? Should an independent third party be invited to build and then lease the MOB to keep the hospital uninvolved? Could this be the physicians?

PART 2

A second problem you face is that of out-migration of potential patients. Many citizens have told you that the hospital is fine for those of lesser economic means, but for those who can afford it, the only health care they will seek is from larger facilities in larger cities. To help fight this problem, the board of directors has given you a mandate to enhance the quality of care. In the board's opinion, you should immediately recruit an anesthesiologist instead of continuing to depend on the three CRNAs. When you tell this to the surgeons, they say, "We have used the

CRNAs for 15 years; we will not use an anesthesiologist." In their best Western vernacular, they tell you, "We are gonna ride the horse that brung us!"

Part 2 Discussion

Will the new anesthesiologist likely be successful if the surgeons remain loyal to the CRNAs? What about other physicians besides the surgeons that could use the anesthesiologist? Could the anesthesiologist perform other anesthesia services besides surgery, such as caring for patients that need pain management services? Could he or she supervise and teach the CRNAs new techniques? Could the hospital add complex new patient services such as open-heart surgery that the CRNAs may not be familiar with or skilled in delivering anesthesia?

PART 3

Finally, the physicians have come to you, requesting that you side with them to request a change in the enabling legislation[a] which created the hospital. In this hospital district, physicians are currently expressly prohibited by law from running for a seat on the board, by the very fact that they are physicians. The hospital's medical staff formally requests that the administrator and hospital support their move to have the legislation changed.

DISCUSSION

Would you want physicians on the Board of Directors? What are the pros and cons of them serving? Do you think anyone in the community or on the current Board of Directors would oppose physicians serving?

---

[a]Hospital districts in this state are created by legislative acts. The act creating the district sets forth what the hospital and its board can and cannot do, how often elections are held, how the administrator is hired, etc. In this case, a seven-person board was created to oversee the hospital, but physicians were specifically prohibited in the original enabling legislative act from serving on the hospital board. To change the enabling legislation, a bill would need to be introduced by a congressional representative and then passed by the legislature and signed by the governor—something not impossible, but of serious nature.

Case 4:

I'm Calling the EEOC and Filing a Complaint

You are the new, female CEO of an 80-bed rural hospital. One of the employees asks if she can speak to you for a moment. Having an open-door policy and wishing to know all the employees, you smile and say, "Of course," and usher her into your office.

She seems a little sheepish and then states, "Speaking woman to woman, I'm sure you'll understand my plight. My department director seems to be attracted to me, and I have continually repelled his advances. He is much older than I am, is not attractive, is married, and frankly, the thought of him irritates me. Moreover, he is not a good boss. I am not trying to get anyone in trouble, but the other night I saw on late-night television a discussion of something called sexual harassment. That is what I think is going on. I am in a hostile work environment, and if he doesn't quit, I'm calling the EEOC and filing a complaint."

DISCUSSION

What steps will you take? What policies should be in place? Will you interview anyone, and if so, whom? If the person who has complained to you chooses to call the EEOC before you investigate, what should you expect and what will you do? Should you call the hospital's attorney? What protection should be afforded the department director?

Case 5:

Controls and Indicators
for the Ship

You are the chief executive officer of a 342-bed acute-care hospital with several clinics. While reflecting on your experiences of the last year, you decide to create a plus and minus column of what you are pleased with and what you have vowed to change.

In the plus column, you realize that you have several solid senior management team members and many competent department directors. Due to the geography of the hospital, you enjoy zero competition; you have good capital equipment and a solid infrastructure. The hospital's reputation in the community is good; in fact, your hospital is viewed as the region's principal medical center.

In the minus column, however, you realize that most of your senior management team, including yourself and the chief medical director, have been reduced to "firefighters." You find yourself constantly jumping from problem area to problem area, never having enough time to enjoy your job, to explore new possibilities, or to visit physicians, government officials, members of the public, or employees You are literally pinned down in your office stomping out fires such as worrying about vendor deliveries on out-of-stock items, dealing with broken equipment, and being responsive to unhappy patients and family members. Many employees are also unhappy, as the recent employee satisfaction survey has demonstrated . . . in short, you are reacting to the environment.

As you begin to consider your options for change, you happen to read an article that states that hospitals are like ocean liners in that there are many departments and operations and all strive to serve the public; in short, you and your management team are the equivalent of the senior leadership of a large cruise ship with you at the helm. This helps you to realize that just like the ship's captain, you cannot be everywhere at the same time, and yet it is critical that you understand what is going on everywhere. What is ahead? Are you approaching an iceberg? Are heavy winds rising? Are the passengers happy? Is the crew about to mutiny?

These thoughts help you and your senior team to realize that you need gauges, instruments, and warning indicators to monitor periodically. You need information that is simple, concise, and that can be trended to understand the ship and what is happening around the ship.

One of your team members suggests that besides macro indicators such as the average daily census, you need micro indicators from each department. When these are reported, it will help you to form a picture to understand when the ship is off course; you want a fixed set of controls and indicators allowing you to be *proactive* and stop problems before they arise, rather than to *react* to problems and continue your firefighting.

DISCUSSION

What do you and your team suggest? What set of macro indicators are you going to monitor? What specific micro indicators do you want your department directors to watch? Why did you select these indicators? How often should these be monitored?

Case 6:

The Case of Jill

Jill is a patient from a local long-term care facility, admitted 2 weeks ago with pneumonia.

Jill is 15 years old, a resident for 12 years of the long-term care facility due to a major head injury when she was 3 years old. She has an extremely low IQ, cannot speak, is blind, and sits either in bed or in a wheelchair, quietly rocking back and forth. Jill's cognitive prognosis is for no change due to the extensive brain damage. She is in the long-term care facility because her father travels extensively and her mother, who is also physically challenged, is unable to care for Jill.

Your hospital has given Jill good care and her pneumonia has subsided. However, the long-term care facility has notified you that they no longer have a bed for Jill; the facility is at capacity and for the near future will not be admitting patients. Jill does not belong in your hospital; she no longer needs acute care, but discharging her to a long-term care facility does not seem to be an option. Home health care is also not an option since Jill needs care for most of the day.

As the social worker and discharge planner think about what to do, they notice that Jill's color has changed and her skin tone appears to be jaundiced. They refer this new problem to Jill's physician who orders a battery of tests. Jill is diagnosed with renal disease and an order for dialysis is written.

When the dialysis needle is placed in Jill's arm, she cries out in pain, lashes out, and is very combative. Since she is blind and doesn't understand the world around her, it is easy to see that her pain is acute, and Jill cannot comprehend what is happening to her.

After three dialysis sessions, Jill's parents come to the hospital at the request of her physician. They are told the following options are open to Jill: 1) she can receive dialysis three times weekly for the next 20 to 30 years because she is otherwise healthy, or 2) the dialysis can be discontinued and Jill would be expected to die within the next 12 months.

After conferring with their minister, Jill's parents decided to discontinue the dialysis treatments. They reason that Jill has a low quality of life and that is not expected to change. The benefits of the treatment are not worth the pain that Jill would have to bear.

Upon learning of the parent's decision, you decide to convene the bioethics committee, who will act as an impartial advisory body. The committee is comprised of you, the CEO; a physician; a nurse; a social worker; the hospital attorney; and one of the committee's volunteer ministers.

Jill's physician objectively presents her case to the committee and the two options that are open. The committee members ask questions and then confer with Jill's parents, who present their views. The committee then decides to confer privately.

As the committee members confer, the hospital's attorney suggests a third option. The state could be contacted and Jill could be removed from the care of her parents. The attorney anticipates that the state would then place Jill in a state institution and would continue to provide dialysis treatment.

DISCUSSION

Discuss Jill's case in detail, as the bioethics committee would; weigh all options. What recommendations do you have?

Case 7:

The Need to Communicate

You are the administrator of a 201-bed acute-care facility located in a medium-sized city somewhere in mid-America. Your hospital provides the normal array of services and you think your management team does a good job. At a suggestion from a staff member, you decide to ask your marketing department to undertake some research. You ask them to form two focus groups to seek perceptions about the hospital. One group should be comprised of a dozen physicians randomly chosen from active medical staff members who have had at least 10 admissions apiece during the past year. The other group, comprised of a dozen citizens, will be acquired by placing, in a large neighborhood supermarket, a recruiting poster seeking paid volunteers. Questions for both groups are open ended and ask for information as to how the hospital is perceived by each group.

After a couple of months, the marketing department prepared the following report:

Summary—Physician Group

This focus group met during lunch with an experienced moderator. They were asked to provide information about the hospital, specifically their chief likes and dislikes. While nearly all voiced the opinion that the facility was up to date, had modern technology, and employed well-trained staff, their chief complaint was that they were never informed of what the hospital was about to undertake, they were always in the dark, and they always felt left out of decision making. To be specific, one physician commented, "I have been on staff for 3 years and wondered what the construction effort was all about at the rear of the hospital. I just found out it is a new outpatient dialysis unit."

Another physician spoke up and complained, "The new CT scanner that was ordered is a Hemotso. If I had known that, I might have persuaded the hospital to switch to Hitachi; it does better spin-echo imaging. It seems that no one ever tells us anything, and we are the ones charged with patient care."

Responses from the remaining physicians were similar.

Summary—Consumer Group

This group of 12 was comprised of 5 men and 7 women of varying ages, all living less than 5 miles from the hospital, 8 having used the hospital within the last 12 months. The focus group was conducted during lunch, the volunteers were paid $50 for their participation, and the group was asked open-ended questions regarding their perceptions of the hospital.

While everyone thought the hospital had the best reputation of any hospital in the city, they all voiced the opinion that they knew little about the hospital. When asked, "What new service provided by the hospital do you feel is the most important?" only one commented about the cardiac cath unit, most could not name *any* new service, and the only other service that was named at all was the emergency department.

You feel disappointed at the perceptions of the two groups, but you also feel this is an opportunity to launch a new and better communication effort, both internally and externally.

DISCUSSION

What do you plan to do to communicate with the physicians and, for that matter, the employees? What do you plan to do to communicate with the public? Please be specific, setting out a strategy, budget, and timetable for each group.

Case 8:

Adding a New Service to the Hospital

It is February 2006 and you are the CEO of a medium sized acute-care medical center. You have been at the hospital for 6 years and are pleased that a Gamma Knife (GK) will be added to the list of services offered by the hospital. In fact, you are expecting the first patient to be scheduled for this procedure about August 2007.

The Gamma Knife is a new procedure for this area of the country. One of your challenges is to inform the public of what the procedure is and how it is done, how it can benefit a patient, the risks involved, and the positive and negative aspects of the surgery.

The hospital's marketing director has just joined the organization from a sales position at Ferrari's of Miami. He is a genius at public relations and marketing, but, in his own words, he "knows zero about health care."

In addition to recruiting the correct personnel to do the procedure, you must lead a team of hospital employees through an integrated approach to the patient, i.e., how the lab, radiology, anesthesia, surgery, ICU, safety, pharmacy, materials management, physical therapy, and the patient education departments can work together for each patient's benefit.

DISCUSSION

Please present steps that you deem appropriate to lead your team of employees toward successful implementation of the GK procedure. You must also build awareness in the public as to the new procedure and who might be candidates for the GK. How will you do this?

Case 9:

The Case of "Baby B"

As you arrive at work on a Monday morning, you find the vice president of nursing, Ms. Pipkin, RN, waiting outside your office with a very worried look, not a usual sign that all went well during the weekend. As the CEO of the hospital, you have relied on her judgment for several years and you think well of her. When she gets upset, you have learned that it is usually more than a simple problem.

Ms. Pipkin opens the dialogue with, "We had a baby taken from the pediatrics ward during the weekend. I didn't beep you or call because the baby was taken by the nurse manager of pediatrics." You quietly compose yourself and ask the nursing vice president to continue.

"Patti is the nurse manager in question. Recently, she and her husband, Tim, were told by their physician that Patti is unable to get pregnant. On Friday night, we had a 14-year-old girl deliver her baby. She then stated to everyone concerned, 'When I leave this hospital I am not taking that baby home with me. Call the state, call anyone you want, but I am leaving the baby here and you can do with it what you want.'"

"Patti is a veteran nurse and is well versed in the law," Ms. Pipkin continued. "Patti understands that the girl, even though only 14, becomes emancipated after giving birth, and legally can sign her baby over to anyone she chooses. Patti found the necessary forms and explained to the girl that she, Patti, would be a very fit parent; she was the nurse manager of pediatrics and understands children very well; and she and her husband, Tim, had wanted children, but just learned that could not have any. With a stroke of a pen, the new mother signed over her baby to Patti and Patti took the baby home on Saturday morning."

You confer with Ms. Pipkin further and then call the hospital's attorney, the local district attorney; the state nursing board, the state hospital association, and the state attorney general's office. After lengthy discussions, each group replies that it can find no rule or statute that has been violated. One person wisecracked that a nurse should not accept gifts from patients, but all declined to become involved because they could see no breach of duty, care, or broken law.

The state attorney general's office tells you that a social study is always done when a couple is given a baby. The state will send a social worker to visit and to assess the potential parents and the environment they provide. If the parents are declared unfit, the baby will be placed in a foster home pending adoption; if they are affirmed fitting, they will be allowed to adopt the baby.

DISCUSSION

Is there an ethical duty on Patti's part not to solicit the baby? How will the community feel about her action? Should the hospital write a new policy regarding this matter? Should the hospital take any action regarding Patti's employment?

Case 10:

The Case of the Relocated Management Team

You and your senior management team have done an extraordinary job in managing the company's medical center in Wisconsin. In fact, on several occasions, the company president has singled you out for special commendations.

One of the company's key regional vice presidents flew into town yesterday and requested an emergency meeting with you and your senior management team. It seems there is a crisis at the company's medical center in Missouri.

In meeting with the vice president, you have learned that the hospital CEO in Missouri has a terminal disease, two of his senior management team members have recently retired, and two others resigned yesterday for other opportunities. There is a critical management vacuum at the top. This has caught the company by surprise and the company has no game plan—in fact, the company president was consulted and suggested to the regional vice president that you and your team be shifted to take over the Missouri facility.

In your meeting with the vice president, she states, "I have confidence in your management abilities and therefore I am reassigning you immediately to the Missouri hospital. You and your team are to report there tomorrow to assume key command and control positions. You will be there for a minimum of 9 months until other staff can be recruited to take your place and you have full authority and responsibility to make any changes you wish. I can tell you that the hospital is 27 percent short of nursing staff, and the contracted pharmacy company that has been managing the pharmacy has give notice that they are leaving in 60 days. On top of that, eight physicians are not renewing their contracts at the end of the year (it is now August 4th); engineering has informed us that the emergency power system is nonoperational and cannot be repaired because it is too old; and the finance director is in jail, charged by the government with embezzling hospital funds for his own personal use."

You also learn in a follow-up meeting that if you do a good job in Missouri, there will be key positions waiting for you and your team in the home office. However, should you fail, the likelihood exists that you will be relocated to the Sand Dune Hospital in Death Valley, a 37-bed facility.

DISCUSSION

What do you think are the central issues for your concern? What do you plan to undertake each month? What information will you immediately request upon arrival? How do you plan to address the employees who you learn were very loyal to the past administration team—many who seem to be contemplating jobs with other hospital companies.

Appendix B
Glossary

Accreditation. A process used by the Joint Commission on Accreditation of Healthcare Organizations (JCAHO) to evaluate the quality of patient care at hospitals and health facilities.

Accredited hospital. A hospital that meets specific operating standards set by the Joint Commission on Accreditation of Healthcare Organizations (JCAHO) or by the American Osteopathic Association. Typically, the seal of accreditation is displayed in the lobby of a hospital.

Admission. The formal acceptance of inpatients into a hospital or other inpatient health facility. Such inpatients are typically provided with room, board, and continuous nursing service and stay at least overnight.

Admitting department. The hospital department that secures patient demographic and financial information on inpatients for registration purposes; schedules preadmission testing; coordinates patient room assignments; records all patient movement including transfers and discharges for the purpose of maintaining accurate census data; and disseminates patient information to other hospital departments.

Advanced directive. Written instructions of a patient's wishes should the patient become incapable of informing the care provider of those wishes.

Advertising. The act or practice of attracting public attention with the specific intent of generating interest or inducing purchase. Advertising is paid for and generally placed in the mass media.

Agency contract nurse. A service referred to as an outside agency that contracts with hospitals to provide registered nurses, licensed practical nurses, and nursing assistants.

Alliance. A formal agreement between several hospitals and/or hospital systems for specific purposes. These arrangements usually operate under a set of bylaws or other written regulations.

Allied health professional. A health worker other than a physician, dentist, podiatrist, or nurse, who is specially trained, and in some cases, licensed, e.g., a physician's assistant. Depending upon the hospital or health facility, this individual may perform tasks that could be performed by a physician. An allied health professional always works under the supervision of a health professional.

Ambulatory care. Medical or health services provided on an outpatient basis. It usually implies the patients are ambulatory and came to the facility for a specific outpatient treatment or service. (Synonym: outpatient care)

Ambulatory care center, freestanding. A facility, not on a hospital campus, offering medical, surgical, diagnostic, and rehabilitative care on an outpatient basis.

Ambulatory hospital. A program based in the hospital or other institution offering intensive medical, psychiatric, nursing, or rehabilitative services to patients during the day hours.

Ambulatory surgery, hospital. Minor elective surgical procedures provided by a hospital on an outpatient basis. By admitting and discharging patients on the day of surgery, such programs reduce hospital costs. (Synonyms: short procedures unit (SPU), same day surgery, come and go surgery, and outpatient surgery)

Ambulatory surgical facility, freestanding. A facility, physically and/or geographically separate and apart from the hospital, which provides surgical treatment to outpatients who do not require overnight hospitalization. Note: Surgical procedures done in offices of private physicians or dentists are not included in this category unless such offices have a distinct area that is used solely for outpatient surgical treatment on a routine, organized basis. (Synonym: freestanding surgi-center)

American College of Healthcare Executives (ACHE). One North Franklin Street, Chicago, Illinois 60606. Formed in 1933. Professional society for hospital and health care managers and executives. It was formerly called the American College of Hospital Administrators (ACHA). The name was changed in 1985.

American Hospital Association (AHA). One Franklin Street, Chicago, Illinois 60606. Formed in 1898. A nationwide association that promotes the public's welfare through the development of better hospital care for all people. The AHA conducts research and educational programs in areas of health care administration, hospital economics, hospital facilities and design, and community relations. In addition, the AHA represents hospitals as a national spokesperson for legislation. The AHA has several separate professional divisions; for example, American Academy of Hospital Attorneys and American Society for Hospital Central Service Personnel. The AHA also offers policy guidance to governmental agencies.

American Medical Association (AMA). 535 Dearborn Street, Chicago, Illinois 60610. Formed in 1847. A nationwide professional association of licensed physicians. Action: Monitors the quality of medical practice. The AMA provides information on drugs, medical therapy, research, food and nutrition, cosmetics and medical quackery; determines the conditions of medical practice and payment; and acts as a watchdog over the growing governmental interest in the nation's health. The AMA also offers policy guidance to governmental agencies.

Americans with Disabilities Act (ADA). 1990 federal act prohibiting discrimination of those with physical disabilities.

Ancillary services. Therapeutic or diagnostic services provided by specific hospital departments (other than nursing service) including but not limited to imaging, laboratories, and anesthesiology. Other (electrocardiograms) ancillary services include but are not limited to respiratory therapy, electroencephalography, heart station, rehabilitative medicine, and pharmacy.

Anesthesiology. The branch of medicine that deals with the administration and study of anesthetics. It involves the administration of local, general, or regional anesthesia before and during surgery.

Anesthesiology department. That hospital department staffed by anesthesiologists and nurse anesthetists who administer anesthesia and anesthetics to patients so that surgical or other authorized procedures may be performed.

Annual report. A yearly publication prepared and issued by a hospital, which details the state of the institution's operations and financial position. Typically, the year's accomplishments, as well as its future plans and programs, are highlighted.

Audit medical and patient care. A periodic and systematic review of quality care within a hospital, usually done by a committee or a designated person following a set process.

Average census. The average number of patients who receive medical or nursing care during a specific reporting period (typically 1 year or month).

Average daily census. The average number of inpatients receiving care each day during a reporting period, excluding newborns. Bed counts of patients are most often done at midnight.

Baccalaureate degree program, nursing. A formal program of study in a 4-year college or university, which educates students in the nursing field. Typically, the college's nursing school provides both classroom and laboratory teaching.

The college's own hospital or its affiliated hospital provides the clinical teaching. Upon graduation from the program, individuals are awarded a bachelor of arts or bachelor of science degree in nursing. Graduates are then eligible to take the state nursing examinations for licensure as registered nurses. (Synonym: bachelor of science in nursing, BSN)

Bad debt. An account, which is uncollectible from a patient, although the patient has or may have the ability to pay. This results in a credit loss for the hospital, clinic, or other health care facility. These losses may be reflected as an allowance from revenue or as an expense of doing business.

Balance sheet. A summary listing of an institution's assets, liabilities, and net worth showing the financial condition of the hospital or business at a specific point in time. For hospitals, net worth is commonly referred to as the fund balance.

Bed. A bed located in a hospital or nursing home used for inpatients. Beds are used as one important measure of an institution's capacity and size.

Bed allocation policy. A hospital's method of assigning inpatient beds. A hospital may establish its own policy. Policies may be established to maximize occupancy or hospital resources; segregate clinical areas—medicine, surgery, obstetrics, and gynecology; minimize bad debts or maximize revenue; and/or to support the hospital's teaching programs (interns and residents) by assigning beds according to teaching needs.

Bed size. The number of hospital beds, vacant or occupied, maintained regularly for use by inpatients during a reporting period (the typical reporting period is 12 months). To determine this amount, first add the total number of beds, which is available every day during the hospital's reporting period. Then, divide this amount by the total number of days in the reporting period. (Synonym: statistical beds)

Bedside telemonitoring equipment. A sophisticated piece of medical equipment used at a patient's bedside for a variety of functions, including recording electrocardiograms, measuring heart and respiratory rates, and recording blood pressure. Although such monitors are equipped with easy-to-use indicators and controls, only medical/nursing personnel who are trained to use the monitor should be responsible for its proper use.

Beeper system. The communications system that medical and health care professionals often use to enable them to stay in touch with the hospital or their office staff. Beeper system is the name given to the radio wave pagers. They can be digital, voice recorders, or a combination of both. Within the hospital, the paging system or beeper system is usually coordinated through the telephone office.

Blood bank. A medical laboratory that collects and types blood from donors then refrigerates the blood until it is needed for transfusions. The unit also analyzes blood from donors to determine compatibility. This process is referred to as "typing" and "crossmatching."

Blood bank technologist. A trained individual, working under the direction of a laboratory director, physician, or pathologist, whose responsibilities include collecting, classifying, storing, and processing of blood, as well as preparing components from whole blood, detecting and identifying antibodies in blood from patients and donors, and selecting and delivering blood suitable for transfusion.

Blue Cross (BC). A private insurance plan that provides coverage for the insured for hospital costs. Most Blue Cross members sign up for coverage at their workplace under a group plan.

Board certified. A professional title of considerable merit awarded to a physician who passes examinations administered by the professional organization that regulates their specialty. The examination cannot be taken until the physician meets requirements established by the specialty board, making them board eligible.

Board of trustees. *See* Governing body.

Bond ratings. General measurements of a bond's quality provided to guide investors in making investments. Bonds that are rated Aaa/AAA are judged to be of the best quality because they carry the smallest degree of investment risk. Bonds are generally rated by one of two companies: Standard & Poor's or Moody's.

Brand name drug. The registered trademark that a manufacturer assigns to one of its drug products. Note: A drug's brand name differs from a drug's generic name, which is the official name by which the drug is known scientifically. Drugs are advertised to physicians chiefly by brand name. (Occasionally, states may have an anti-substitution law, which forbids a pharmacist from substituting a physician's prescription for a brand name drug with either an equivalent brand name drug or a generic drug made by a different manufacturer, even though either of the substitutions may be less expensive than the prescribed drugs.) (Synonyms: trade name, patent name)

Budget. The dollar amounts required to meet a hospital's immediate administrative objectives, as well as its operation and financing plans for a given time period, usually a year. It is the hospital's plan for that period expressed in dollars and cents.

Budget, cash. The details of a business's or hospital's anticipated receipts and cash disbursements for a forthcoming budget period. It is usually used to forecast the need for cash to meet operating expenses and to determine the amount of cash that will be available for capital purchases, acquisitions, and investing.

Business office manager. That individual who supervises and coordinates the operations of a hospital's business office, including the supervision of office functions, such as bookkeeping, typing, clerical services, word processing, record keeping, files, and reports in accordance with hospital standards.

Bylaws. The rules, regulations, and ordinances enacted by a given organization to provide the basis for its own self-government. In a hospital, two major sets of bylaws are the governing body bylaws, or hospital bylaws, and the medical staff bylaws.

Capital budget. A financial plan detailing anticipated capital expenditures principally for equipment (medical and nonmedical) and building renovation and construction. The sources of these funds are identified as part of the capital budget. Potential sources are operating funds, restricted funds, and outside financing such as leases or debt finances and fund-raising.

Cardiac Care Unit (CCU). A specialized cardiac unit reserved for observation and recovery of patients who have undergone an intensive cardiac procedure or who have critical cardiac problems (e.g., heart attacks). Units are equipped with electrocardiographic and hemodynamic monitoring equipment.

Certification. The process by which a government or private agency or a health-related association evaluates and recognizes individual, institutional, or educational programs in meeting predetermined standards.

Certified laboratory assistant (CLA). Individuals who perform routine clinical laboratory procedures and work under the supervision of a medical technologist or pathologist.

Chief executive officer (CEO). The individual responsible for the overall management of the hospital. An individual appointed by the governing body to assure that the mission and goals of the institution are carried out as determined by the bylaws of the hospital. The job includes planning, organizing, and directing all hospital activities in accordance with objectives and policies established by the board, developing ongoing and future hospital programs, presenting annual budgets, planning, and implementing sound organizational plans. (Synonyms: administrator, president, hospital administrator, hospital director, superintendent)

Chief financial officer (CFO). The individual responsible for an organization's overall financial plans and policies along with the administration of accounting practices. The job includes directing the hospital's treasury, budgeting, audit, tax, and accounting functions, and it may include the purchase of real estate. Specific responsibilities include developing and coordinating all necessary and appropriate accounting and statistical data with and for all the departments.

Chief operating officer (COO). The second highest management position in the hospital. He/she is responsible for the management of day-to-day internal hospital operations. In the absence of the chief executive officer, the chief operating officer is responsible for managing the hospital. (Synonyms: assistant administrator, executive vice-president, senior vice president)

Children's hospital. This is a specialty hospital, specializing in inpatient and outpatient care, limited to the treatment of diseases and injuries of children.

Chronic illness. Any illness that has continued for a long period and may recur in the future. Alterations in such illnesses are slow.

Clinic. An independent organization of physicians and allied health personnel or a hospital-operated facility designed to provide preventive, diagnostic, therapeutic, rehabilitative, or palliative services on an outpatient basis.

Clinical engineer. A professional with an associate or bachelor of science degree in biomedical engineering. This individual utilizes engineering techniques to repair or develop equipment, instruments, processes, and systems for the medical care of patients and the overall maintenance and improvement of health care systems. Some biomedical engineers develop lasers, pacemakers, and artificial organs such as hearts and kidneys. Others adapt computer systems to hospital systems to increase operating efficiency. Typically, they work in hospitals, private medically related industries, or medical settings (Synonym: biomedical engineer)

Clinical nurse specialist. A registered nurse with both a master's degree and clinical expertise in a clinical area (e.g., surgical, critical care, medicine, or cardiology).

Clinical outcomes. A form of medical and/or nursing evaluation involving the measurement of the patient care process against criteria such as the status of the patient at discharge.

Community hospital. A hospital that is established to meet the medical and health needs of a specific geographic area. Usually these hospitals are nonprofit, but they may be proprietary, for profit. Community hospitals are generally nonfederal, short-term, and general care hospitals.

Comprehensive outpatient rehabilitation facility (CORF). A facility providing comprehensive outpatient rehabilitation services, including physician's services, physical therapy, occupational therapy, speech-language pathology, respiratory therapy, prosthetic supplies, and home environment evaluation. These services are reimbursable under Medicare Part B.

Computerized axial tomography (CAT). A radiographic technique more sensitive than conventional x-ray systems in detecting variations among soft tissues with similar densities. It provides highly detailed, cross-sectional, three-dimensional pictures, which, because they are thin slices or cross sections of the body, establish more precisely than conventional x-rays the area and depth of the abnormality. (Synonym: CAT scan)

Consent forms. The documents that patients are asked to sign giving permission to the hospital or its physicians to perform procedures during the patient's hospital stay, whether as an outpatient or inpatient. There are two general types of consent forms, one that details their general treatment and diagnosis and the other one for special medical or surgical procedures. The most important element in the issue of consent is that the physician in the hospital clearly explains the procedures to be performed to the patient and obtains the patient's consent to the procedures. This is known as an informal consent form.

Continuing medical education (CME). Postgraduate education aimed at maintaining, updating, and extending a physician's knowledge and skills. Many professional organizations and state licensing boards require a physician to participate in CME activities.

Contract management. A system whereby hospital management contracts with an outside management company to provide certain management services, e.g., dietary, housekeeping, and data processing services. It is also possible to employ contract management for the total management of a hospital. (Synonym: contract service)

Controller. The hospital position responsible for the traditional financial activities of the hospital, including general accounting, reimbursement, and budgeting. In smaller institutions, this position may also be the chief financial officer (CFO). In larger institutions, the controller reports to a CFO.

Corporate compliance committee. A hospital-wide committee designed to regularly audit and insure that the hospital is in compliance with all federal, state, and local laws.

Corporate restructuring. The regrouping of a hospital's corporate hierarchy by creating holding companies or foundations in order to guard assets, provide flexibility for diversification, accomplish a broader mission, increase effectiveness, and permit capital accumulation. (Synonym: corporate reorganization)

Cost reimbursement. Payment to hospitals and other providers by a third-party carrier for costs actually incurred by the providers; cost rates are calculated after the service is rendered.

Cost reports. The cost-analysis documents prepared by a health care facility to be submitted to third-party payers as part of contract agreements. These reports are used as the basis for cost reimbursement.

Credentials committee. A medical staff committee that interviews and reviews credentials and delineation of privileges for each new medical staff applicant.

Darling case. A landmark legal case, *Darling v. Charleston Community Hospital*, found that the hospital was responsible to oversee and monitor the quality and process of medical care in the institution, and that these functions were not exclusively the responsibility of the medical staff.

Delinquent medical records. Those inpatient medical records not completed within a given time period, usually 15 to 30 days following the patient's discharge.

Development office. That section of the hospital responsible for directing, planning, and coordinating direct fund-raising activities and programs for the hospital. This section may also be responsible for the hospital's public relations activities. (Synonym: fund-raising office)

Diagnostic related group (DRG) rate. A dollar amount used by Medicare to pay hospitals for services rendered. It is based on the average of all patients belonging to a specific DRG adjusted for economic factors, inflation, and bad debts.

Dietary department. That hospital department equipped, designed, and staffed to prepare food to meet the normal and therapeutic nutritional needs of the patients and hospital staff. (Synonym: food service department)

Dietician. A professional, educated and trained to deal with the scientific aspects of human nutrition and diets. The dietician develops specific food and nutritional plans for patients.

Diploma school of nursing. A 2- to 3-year professional nursing program generally affiliated with a hospital, which leads to a diploma.

Director of nurses. Old term for the current term of vice president of nursing services.

Discharge planning. The planning and organization process undertaken by a committee of a hospital medical staff that addresses patient discharges into the community, home, or appropriate health care facilities. This process begins at the time of admission or, in elective cases, prior to admission.

Elective admission. The admission of a patient to a hospital prior to the actual scheduled date of admission. This admission can be delayed without potential risk to the health of the individual.

Electrocardiography (EKG). A cardiac procedure used at the heart station to diagnose irregularities in heart action. It records changes in electrical current during a heartbeat, providing an important source of medical diagnostic information.

Electroencephalography (EEG). A procedure used to measure the brain's electrical signals. This is useful in diagnosing epilepsy, brain tumors, strokes, and other metabolic abnormalities.

Emergency admission. The admission of a patient to a hospital immediately or within a very short period of time in order to save the patient's life or to protect the patient's health and well-being. Other general categories of admission are urgent, usually requiring admission within 12–24 hours, or elective, when a patient can wait for admission without any adverse effects.

Emergency center, freestanding (FEC). A facility structured, equipped, and staffed to offer primary, urgent, and emergency services. These facilities often offer laboratory and radiographic services as well, and often have transfer agreements with area hospitals for sending severely ill patients needing hospitalization to the hospital once the patients are stable.

Emergency department (ED). That department or unit of a hospital organized to provide medical services necessary to sustain life or to prevent critical consequences. This area sometimes provides nonurgent, walk-in care. The department is usually staffed 24 hours per day by physicians and nurses. (Synonym: emergency service)

Emergency Medical Treatment and Active Labor Act (EMTALA). A major law assuring patients presenting to an emergency department of at least being stabilized and/or transferred.

Emergency patient. An outpatient, usually acutely ill, who uses a hospital or freestanding emergency department for treatment.

Employment Retirement Income Security Act (ERISA). A 1974 federal act protecting employee benefits.

Equal Employment Opportunity Commission (EEOC). Federal agency in charge of administrative and judicial enforcement of the federal civil rights laws which prohibit discrimination based on age, race, color, religion, sex, or natural origin.

Equal Pay Act. Federal act prohibiting pay differences between men and women doing the same work.

Executive committee. The senior committee of a governing body (hospital board or medical staff) It may also be the ruling body.

Expenses. The sum of all incurred costs for services used or consumed in performing some activity during a given time period and from which no benefit will exist beyond the stated period.

Fair Labor Standards Act. Law that sets nationwide minimum wages and maximum hours.

Fiduciary. A person who undertakes a solemn duty to act for the benefit of another, under a given set of circumstances (e.g., the members of the governing body of a hospital have a fiduciary responsibility to the community).

Financial statements. Summaries of the financial activities of a hospital or other business. The balance sheet includes itemized listings of the hospital's assets and liabilities and the net worth of the hospital. The income statement, or profit and loss statement, lists the hospital's income or revenue and its expenses or costs.

Fluoroscopy. Technique used to view the body structure by sending x-rays through the body part to be examined and then observing the shadows cast on a glaring screen.

Formulary. A listing of drugs, usually by their generic names, intended to include sufficient range of medicines to enable a physician or dentist to prescribe medically appropriate treatment for all reasonable common illnesses. A formulary may also be a listing of drugs for which a third party will or will not pay.

Full time equivalent (FTE). The term used in hospital budgeting and human resources that represents the number of worked hours that a full-time employee would be expected to work in a given year. In other words, 40 hours a week or 2,080 annual hours. This term is used in hospital budgeting, position control and productivity.

General fund/fund accounting. Technique that accounts for separate entities in a hospital fund. The account group used to record transactions arising out of general operations in the day-to-day financial and operational activities of the hospital. (Synonym: hospital accounting)

Generic drug. The official scientific name for a drug.

Governing body. A hospital's ruling body, responsible for the institution's overall operation. Its essential functions include defining objectives, mandating policies, maintaining the programs and resources necessary to implement policies, and monitoring progress to guarantee the policy objectives are met. In addition, it hires the hospital's CEO. Note: The Board of Trustees should not be mistaken for the lay advisory board. (Synonyms: the board, board of directors, board of trustees, board of governors)

Graduate nurse (GN). A nurse who has graduated from an approved program of professional nursing but who has not yet received the registered nurse (RN) licensure.

Group practice. A formal association of physicians providing either specialty or comprehensive medical care on an outpatient basis. (Synonyms: single specialty group, general practice group, multispecialty group)

Group purchasing. An arrangement where a group of hospitals band together, often through a third party, e.g., the group purchaser, in order to purchase goods and services at the lowest price because the arrangement makes it feasible for them to engage in quantity purchasing. (Synonym: shared purchasing)

Health administration. The management of resources, procedures, and systems operating to meet the needs and wants of a health care system. (Synonyms: health care administration, hospital administration)

Health Insurance Portability and Accountability Act (HIPAA). This federal act, passed in 1996, assures portability of health insurance, adds enforcement to health care fraud and abuse, enforces standards for health care, and guarantees security and privacy of health information.

Health maintenance organization (HMO). Third-party payer plans. There are two fundamental types of HMO plans: (1) the group model, where HMOs contract with several group practices and share the risk of the venture with the physicians; and (2) independent practice associations (IPAs), loose-knit, prepaid plans that contract with individual physicians to treat patients in their offices, often on a fee-for-service basis.

Health system. The organization of human resources, facilities, and medical technology. (Synonym: medical system)

Heart Diagnostics (or less common, older term, Heart Station). That unit or section of a hospital that coordinates cardiac tests and procedures. Some may be done on an outpatient basis (e.g., EKGs).

Hill-Burton Act. The legislative act that led to federal legislation and programs offering federal support for construction and modernization of hospitals and other health facilities. This program began with Public Law 79-725, The Hospital Survey and Construction Act of 1946, and has been amended often.

Home care nurse. A registered nurse (preferably with a BSN and 2 years of hospital experience) who intermittently visits patients at their homes to carry out a nursing care plan approved by a physician. Typical duties include injections, incision care, rehabilitation activities, patient education, and other skilled care. (Synonym: visiting nurse)

Home health care. A formal program offering medical and nursing care, therapeutic services, and social services to patients in their homes. (Synonym: home care services)

Hospice care. A program providing palliative and supportive care for terminally ill patients and their families either directly or on a consulting basis with the patient's physician or another community agency. Emphasis is placed on system control, preparation for death, and support of the survivors. A hospice program may be housed and based in a facility such as a hospital, or it may be a freestanding hospice.

Hospital. An institution producing medical and health care every day around the clock. Its primary function is to provide inpatient and outpatient services, including diagnostic and therapeutic services, for a variety of medical and surgical conditions. Some also provide emergency care. Hospitals can be teaching or nonteaching, specialty or nonspecialty (psychiatric, general, etc.), proprietary (for-profit) or not-for-profit (government, local, private) entities. The majority of hospitals in the United States are short-term acute-care, general, and non-profit.

Hospital bylaws. The guidelines, rules, and regulations governing the actions and regulating the affairs of a hospital governing board.

Hospital chaplains. Members of the clergy who provide religious minister and pastoral care and services to patients, their families, and members of the hospital staff.

Hospitalist. Physician caring only for hospitalized patients; usually provides care to other physicians' patients.

Hospital ledger. An accounting record detailing the various accounts in a hospital categorized into assets, liabilities, revenues, and expenses. Entries are made into this document periodically (generally monthly) from various journals. The general ledger allows for financial analysis over a long period.

Human resources. The hospital department responsible, in conjunction with other hospital departments, for recruitment, selection, orientation, and employee training programs. The department is also responsible for maintaining personnel records and statistics, initiating and maintaining salary and wage administration, and recommending personnel policy and procedure to the hospital administrator. (Synonym: personnel department)

Incident report. A written report detailing an accident or error in the care of a patient. Hospitals require the nurse and/or the physician in charge to complete the form as soon as possible following the accident to ensure accuracy. (Synonym: accident report)

Income statement of revenue and expenses. A summary of the operations of a hospital in terms of revenue generated from patient services and other sources and the expenses incurred to render those services. (Synonyms: profit and loss statement, income statement)

Independent laboratory. A freestanding laboratory not affiliated with any physician's office or hospital.

Infection control. The process of identification, control, and prevention of hospital-acquired (nosocomial) infections. This is usually a responsibility of a hospital medical staff committee with the support of and in conjunction with an infection control practitioner.

Infection control committee. That hospital or medical staff committee responsible for overseeing the infection control activities in the institution. The committee usually consists of representatives from the medical staff, the clinical laboratory, administration, nursing staff, and, at times, the housekeeping department.

Informed consent. Consent given by a patient for a proposed medical treatment or procedure after a physician has explained things that a reasonable person would consider material to decision making, such as the treatment or procedure, the risks involved, as well as alternatives available.

Inpatient. A patient who has been admitted for at least one night to a hospital or other health facility for the purpose of receiving diagnostic treatment or other medical service.

Inpatient component. An element of the hospital-medical care system characterized by the hospital bed. (Synonym: hospital component)

Intensive care unit (ICU). A special medical and nursing section of a hospital with extensive monitoring and treatment equipment, allowing minute-to-minute observation and treatment of critically ill or injured patients.

Intermediate care facility (ICF). An institution or distinct part of an institution providing nursing care or rehabilitative services to patients who do not require inpatient hospital care.

Intern. A graduate of a medical or dental school enrolled in the first year of post-graduate education in an accredited training program, usually in a hospital. (Synonym: postgraduate year, first-year resident)

Internship (medical). A period of on-the-job training for physicians and other health professionals, usually lasting 1 year and occurring just after graduation from medical school.

Investor-owned hospital. A privately owned medical facility operating for profit. (Synonym: proprietary hospital)

Job description. A summary of the key features, elements, or requirements of a specific job category. This summary is generally written after a review of the job, called a job analysis.

Joint Commission International (JCI). Begun by JCAHO in 1999, it provides accreditation surveys and standards for international health care organizations.

Joint Commission on the Accreditation of Health Care Organizations (JCAHO). 875 North Michigan Avenue, Chicago, Illinois 60611. Formed in 1951. A private, nonprofit organization that traces its beginnings to the American College of Surgeons but now involves other professional associations including the American Hospital Association, the American Medical Association and the American College of Physicians. Its purpose is to establish minimum standards of quality care and operations for hospitals. Hospitals voluntarily request a survey for accreditation. Most hospitals seek it since many other issues, such as state licensure, third-party reimbursement, internships and residencies, as well as expansion of facilities are contingent upon receiving accreditation.

Joint venture. An organization or association formed by two or more parties for a single purpose or undertaking. Such an organization may make its membership liable for the organization's debts.

Laboratory department. That unit or department in a hospital or health care facility staffed, equipped, and designed to perform clinical tests and procedures through detailed analysis and examination of specimens. The laboratory is usually divided into sections, including anatomical pathology, clinical chemistry, cytopathology, hematology, and microbiology. (Synonyms: clinical laboratory, laboratory service, medical laboratory, laboratory, lab)

Laboratory report. A document identifying the results of diagnostic tests in a clinical laboratory. Such reports, requested by a physician, are generally used to determine baseline clinical data on a patient or to determine a patient's diagnosis.

Length of stay (LOS). The time an inpatient remains in a hospital or other health facility from date of admission to date of discharge.

Length of stay, average. The average number of days of service rendered to each patient who is discharged during a given time period. To compute this figure, divide the total number of days spent in the hospital by patients discharged in a given time period by the total number of inpatients discharged during the time period. Example: 120 total patient days for 20 patients discharged. The average length of stay is 120/20 = 6 days.

Licensure. Permission granted to an individual or organization by competent authority, usually public, enabling the individual or organization to engage in a practice, occupation, or activity that, without permission, is unlawful.

Long-range plan. A corporate or managerial plan for the operation and functioning of a hospital or institution for the long term, usually 3 to 10 years, including any planned changes in services to be provided, service areas, and proposed buildings or remodeling plans. (Synonym: corporate strategy)

Long-term care. Health and medical care and social services provided on a continual basis to patients suffering from chronic medical and mental conditions.

Long-term care facilities. A range of institutions that provide various levels of long-term care including maintenance and/or nursing care to people who are unable to care for themselves, many of whom have health problems ranging from minimal to severe. Such facilities primarily provide care for patients with long-term illnesses or low prospects for recovery that require regular medical assessment and continuous nursing care. This term includes freestanding institutions or other identifiable components of health care facilities providing nursing care and related services, as well as personal care and residential care. (Synonyms: nursing home, intermediate care facilities, skilled nursing facilities)

Magnetic resonance imaging (MRI). A diagnostic procedure using large magnets and radio signals to produce tomography images of a patient's anatomical structures. This diagnostic tool also has the capability of evaluating a patient's chemical disturbances at the cellular level. The older (original) term for this was nuclear magnetic resonance (NMR).

Maintenance department. That unit, division, or department in a hospital responsible for repair and servicing of a hospital's physical plant, including the hospital grounds, buildings, and equipment. It may also include the provision, distribution, and monitoring of water, light, heat, power, and other building service systems throughout the physical plant.

Malpractice. The professional misconduct or lack of ordinary skill in the performance of a professional act. A professional is liable for the damages or injuries caused by his/her malpractice. When applied to a health practitioner, it is called medical malpractice.

Malpractice suit. Legal proceeding by a plaintiff seeking enforcement of his rights for malpractice.

Management information system (MIS). System that collects data from many areas of a hospital to provide all levels of hospital management with timely, meaningful information on hospital operations.

Market research. The planning, obtaining, display, and analysis of data related to the marketing of a product/service to fulfill a company's mission and objectives.

Marketing. A system of planning, promoting, and distributing needed and wanted services to both present and potential customers. A hospital's customers can include physicians, patients, insurance companies, or employers.

Marketing audit. A marketing tool providing an extensive view of a hospital's or a business's services, its image, and its market segments.

Marketing plan/program. The process of presenting products/services to the marketplace including product definition, product location or place, product price, and product promotion, including public relations and advertising.

Medicaid (MA). A federal health insurance plan, authorized by Title XIX of the Social Security Act, Public Law 89-97, administered by individual states to provide health care for the poor. (Synonym: medical assistance program)

Medical College Admission Test (MCAT). A standardized test required or strongly recommended by nearly all US medical schools as part of the admissions process. Results of this test are evaluated by the medical schools' admissions committees to determine a student's ability to handle medical school course work.

Medical director. The physician on the hospital medical staff who is either appointed by the board, elected by the medical staff, or employed by the institution to serve as the medical administrative head of medical staff affairs. If a physician is elected by the medical staff, he/she may be called the president of the medical staff. (Synonym: chief of staff)

Medical office building (MOB). A building either freestanding or attached to a hospital where a physician or other health practitioner can establish an office. An MOB is sometimes used as a marketing tool for hospitals to attract and retain physicians.

Medical record. Patient's file containing sufficient information to identify clearly the patient, to justify the patient's diagnosis and treatment, and to document accurately the results. The record serves as a basis for planning and continuity of patient care and provides a means of communication among physicians and any other professionals involved in the patient's care. The record also serves as a basis for review, study, and evaluation on serving and protecting the legal interests of the patient, hospital, and responsible practitioner. The content of each record is usually confidential. The record is the property of the hospital; however, others may have access to the record with signed release from the patient. (Synonym: chart, medical chart)

Medical records, department of. That hospital department responsible for the cataloging, maintenance, processing, and control of patient hospital medical records. This unit may be responsible for the statistical and qualitative preparation and analysis of the information in the medical record to aid in the evaluation of patient care. The department prepares records subpoenaed by the courts and interprets medical-legal aspects of records to protect the interests of the hospital.

Medical school. An institution for higher learning accredited by the Association of American Medical Colleges. Medical colleges are accredited to provide courses in arts and science of medicine and related subjects and are empowered to grant an academic degree in medicine.

Medical staff appointment. The appointment by the hospital board of trustees of a physician or dentist to a hospital's medical staff based on the approval of the credentials committee of the medical staff. Appointment includes delineation of clinical privileges. There are different categories of medical staff membership: active, courtesy, consulting, and honorary.

Medical staff, attending. A category of a hospital's medical staff including physicians and dentists who contribute actively to the hospital by admitting and caring for patients on a regular basis. The medical staff might also include other practitioners including podiatrists. These individuals are eligible to vote and hold office in the medical staff organization.

Medical staff bylaws. A document required by the Joint Commission on the Accreditation of Hospitals Healthcare Organizations (JCAHO) outlining the activities, functions, roles, purpose, rules, and regulations of a hospital's medical staff. The bylaws identify and define the key operating committees of the medical staff and their functions.

Medical students. Individuals enrolled in an accredited medical school studying to become physicians.

Medical technologist. An individual trained in the use of clinical laboratory equipment to test human body tissues and fluids, culture bacteria to identify organisms causing disease, analyze blood factors, and trace cancer with radionuclides. Medical technologists specialize in blood banking microbiology, chemistry, and nuclear medical technology.

Medicare. Title XVIII of the Social Security Act, Public Law 89-97. A federal program that pays providers for certain medical and other health services for individuals 65 years of age or older or the disabled, regardless of their income. The program has two parts: hospital insurance (Part A) and medical insurance (Part B). Part B is also known as supplementary medical insurance (SMI).

Merger. The resulting condition after one business, corporation, or hospital secures the capital stock of another business. The merged corporation's stock is usually then dissolved.

Morbidity and mortality committee. Hospital committee that reviews unusual deaths and patterns in death.

Morgue. That area in a hospital where patients who have died are housed. It is usually connected to an autopsy room.

Multihospital system. A central association that owns and/or leases or controls, by contract, two or more hospitals. Some of the benefits of such a system are easier availability of capital markets, mutual purchasing for greater economies of scale, and mutual use of technical and management personnel. There are two types of multihospital systems: not-for-profit (which includes church-affiliated) or investor-owned, for profit. (Synonym: multis)

Narcotics and barbiturates. Medications that are under the control of the Drug Enforcement Administration (DEA). (Synonym: controlled substances)

National Resident Matching Program. Official plan and process for placement of medical school graduates into their first year of graduate medical education. The program matches the preferences of medical students for certain internships and residencies with available hospital positions. The matching process is carried out under complete confidentiality. It is frequently called "the match."

Not-for-profit hospital. An institution defined as a nonproprietary hospital. Not-for-profit hospitals include state and local government-owned facilities. (Synonym: voluntary hospital)

Nuclear medicine. The field of medicine concerned with the diagnostic, therapeutic, and investigative use of radioactive compounds. Sometimes it is considered a subspecialty of radiology.

Nurse. A registered nurse (RN) or licensed practical nurse (LPN). The term usually refers to an RN, who has more education and responsibility than an LPN.

Nurse manager. The registered nurse responsible and accountable for the total operation of one single nursing unit 24 hours a day, 7 days a week. The nurse manager supervises the personnel in this patient care unit, is accountable for the quality of the nursing care on the unit, controls the supplies and material for the unit, and usually schedules the nursing staff in the unit. Generally, nurse managers have a staff of nurses working for them. (Synonym: nurse manager, patient care manager)

Nurse scheduling. The process in nursing management of determining when and what nursing personnel will be on duty each shift. The schedule usually applies for a specified period (4 to 6 weeks) and is tailored to each individual nursing unit's needs. The needs are often determined by a patient classification or acuity system.

Nurse staffing. The process in nursing management primarily concerned with scheduling the correct amount of nursing hours needed to staff adequately a particular nursing unit.

Nurses' station. That part of a nursing unit serving as the section focal point of administration, record keeping, and communication. Often this is where patient records for the entire nursing unit are kept.

Nursing. The act of providing nursing care to patients, their families, and, in the broader sense, communities. Some nursing care activities may be performed by licensed practical nurses and nurses' aides. The hospital nursing function is organized under a nursing service department, headed by a director of nursing or vice president of nursing.

Nursing, primary care. A system in which a professional nurse, in collaboration with other members of a nursing team, assumes responsibility and accountability for total care of a group of patients.

Nursing service department. That department responsible for providing nursing care to meet patients' physical and psychological needs and to collaborate with patients' physicians in developing and implementing patient treatment plans.

Nursing staffing standard. A standard providing a frame of reference for proper nurse staffing on a patient unit. These staffing standards are usually expressed in terms of nursing hours per patient day. (Synonym: nursing norm)

Nursing supervisor. A registered nurse who supervises or directs the activities of two or more nursing units. A nursing supervisor usually manages and directs the nursing services activities during the evenings, nights, and weekends. (Synonym: patient care coordinator)

Nursing, team. A team composed of registered or graduate nurses, practical nurses, aides, and orderlies providing bedside nursing care to a group of patients under the supervision of a team leader who is a registered nurse.

Nursing unit. That geographical section, division, or area of a hospital at which the nursing organization functions. In hospitals, these geographic divisions are often located on nursing or patient floors and may be arranged along medical/surgical specialty lines. The nursing personnel in charge of these units are called nurse managers. They report to a nursing supervisor or assistant director of nursing, or in some cases, directly to the director of nursing. While there is a variety of sizes and shapes of nursing units, most have somewhere between 20 and 40 inpatient beds.

Occupancy rate. A measure of inpatient hospital use. The ratio of inpatient beds occupied to inpatient beds available for occupancy.

Occupational Safety and Health Administration (OSHA). Federal agency established by a 1970 act to ensure all employees in the United States have a safe and healthful workplace.

Occupational therapist (OT). A registered professional trained to work with individuals who have experienced physical injuries or illnesses, psychological or developmental problems, or problems associated with the aging process. An OT requires a bachelor's degree in occupational therapy.

Operating budget. A financial plan detailing estimated income and expenses for a given time period, usually a fiscal year. Proposed income is classified by revenue sources; proposed expenses are accounted for by natural classification, such as salaries, benefits, and supplies.

Osteopath (DO). A physician similar to an MD but who has graduated from a school of osteopathic medicine.

Outpatient. A patient receiving ambulatory care at a hospital or other health facility without being admitted as an inpatient.

Outpatient department. An organized unit of a hospital where outpatient services are delivered. This would include general and specialty hospital clinics.

Outreach. The process by which a hospital interacts with its surrounding communities. This may involve meeting community or patient needs, locating new services within the community, or offering educational health and wellness programs in addition to medical care programs. Hospitals may assign personnel to work in outreach activities.

Parent company. A separate corporate and legal entity/organization used by health care organizations for a variety of reasons, among them to react to opportunities in the marketplace. Hospitals form holding companies by a process of corporate reorganization. (Synonyms: holding company, foundation)

Part A of Medicare. Refers to the Title XVIII of Health Insurance for the Aged of the Society Security Act, Public Law 89-97, which became effective July 1, 1966, and applies to services rendered by a provider (e.g., hospital) to an eligible beneficiary. This part is commonly referred to as hospital insurance.

Part B of Medicare. Refers to Title XVIII of Health Insurance for the Aged of the Social Security Act, Public Law 89-97, which became effective July 1, 1966, and applies to services rendered by a physician to an eligible beneficiary. This part is commonly referred to as supplementary medical insurance.

Pathological services. Services performed in both clinical and anatomical pathology including microbiological, serological, chemical, hematological, biophysical, cytological, immunohematological, and pathological examinations performed on materials derived from the human body. These examinations provide information for the diagnosis, prevention, or treatment of a disease or assessment of a medical condition. (Synonyms: pathology department, clinical laboratories)

Patient accounts and billing department. The department (traditionally referred to as the business office) responsible for managing patient accounts, hospital receivables, and patient bills.

Pathological services. Services performed in both clinical and anatomical pathology including microbiological, serological, chemical, hematological, biophysical, cytological, immunohematological, and pathological examinations performed on materials derived from the human body. These examinations provide information for the diagnosis, prevention, or treatment of a disease or assessment of a medical condition. (Synonyms: pathology department, clinical laboratories)

Patient accounts and billing department. The department (traditionally referred to as the business office) responsible for managing patient accounts, hospital receivables, and patient bills.

Patient day. A unit of measure denoting room and board facilities and services provided during one 24-hour period to an inpatient. The numbers of such days in a month are called patient days per month.

Patient representative. An individual who works with patients, their families, hospital departments and staff, medical staff, and administration in investigating patient complaints and problems with a patient's hospital care. (Synonym: ombudsman)

Patient's Bill of Rights. An outline of the treatment and care a patient has the right to expect during hospitalization. The American Hospital Association has furnished a 12-point bill of rights as a guideline to hospitals that the hospitals can modify to accommodate local laws or customs.

Pediatric unit. A hospital clinical care unit with facilities, equipment, and personnel for the care of infants, children, and adolescents, excluding obstetrical and newborn care.

Peer review organization (PRO). A federally funded organization established by the Social Security Act of 1983 that performs utilization and quality review in order to monitor hospitals and physicians. The organization also monitors all health care services provided to Medicare beneficiaries. Peer review organizations replaced the professional standards review organizations (PSROs) established in 1972. Recently renamed Quality Improvement Organization (QIO).

Pharmacy. The art, science, and practice of preparing, preserving, compounding and dispensing drugs, as well as giving appropriate instructions for and monitoring their use. Also a location (place) where pharmaceuticals are prepared and dispensed. (Synonym: apothecary)

Pharmacy and therapeutic committee. A committee of hospital medical staff personnel concerned with the development and monitoring of pharmacy and

Physician. Any individual with a medical doctorate degree, MD or DO.

Physician's assistant (PA). An individual who extends the service of a supervising physician by taking medical histories, performing physical examinations, and in circumscribed areas, diagnosing and treating patients.

Polygraph Protection Act. Federal law prohibiting most employers from subjecting employees to lie detector examinations.

Preadmission certification. Review and approval of the necessity and appropriateness for proposed inpatient service. The term also refers to actual admission to an institution prior to the proposed admission time.

Preadmission testing (PAT). Diagnostic tests performed in hospital outpatient areas prior to a patient's admission to the hospital. This system is used to verify the need for a hospital admission and/or reduce the inpatient's length of stay.

Preferred provider arrangement (PPA). A direct contractual arrangement among hospitals, physicians, insurers, employers, or third-party administrators in which providers join together to offer health care for a distinct group of people. These contracts normally have three distinguishing features in common: discounts from standard charges, monetary goals for single subscribers (insurers) to utilize contracting providers, and broad utilization review programs. (Synonym: preferred provider organization)

Pregnancy Discrimination Act. A federal act protecting pregnant women from discrimination based on their pregnancy.

Private practice. A medical practice wherein both the practitioner and the practice are independent of any external policy control.

Privileges, clinical. A permission granted to physicians and selected other practitioners, enabling them to render specific diagnostic, therapeutic, medical, dental, podiatric, or surgical services within the hospital.

Privileged communication. Statements made to a physician, attorney, spouse, or anyone else in a position of trust. Such communication is protected by law and cannot be revealed without the permission of the parties involved.

Professional standards review organization (PSRO). An organization created by the Social Security Amendments of 1972 which the then Department of Health, Education and Welfare charged with the responsibility of operating professional review systems to determine whether hospital services were medically necessary, provided properly, carried out on a timely basis, and met with professional standards. It was conceived as a nationwide network of locally based physicians' groups. It was disbanded in 1983 due to excessive operating costs and little documented impact on patient care.

Prospective payment system (PPS). A method of payment to hospitals in which rates for services are established in advance based on a DRG system or some other methodology.

Psychiatric hospital. A specialty institution primarily concerned with providing inpatient and outpatient care and treatment for the mentally ill.

Public relations (PR). Developing goodwill with specific publics. In the hospital, the public can include patients, physicians, employees, business and industry, and the community.

Purchasing department. That department of a hospital responsible for the evaluation and procurement of the institution's supplies and specified equipment. (Synonym: procurement department)

Quality care. The degree to which patient care services increase the probability of desired patient outcomes.

Quality improvement (QA). Actions taken to assure quality medical and nursing care. Third-party payers and agencies frequently initiate, encourage, or mandate the establishment of such programs.

Quality improvement program (QIP). An institutional program that generally involves a continuous process and regular review of the quality of patient care provided by the institution.

Radiation therapy. A form of medical treatment using ionizing radiation to destroy cancer and other tumors or neoplasm with minimal damage to surrounding healthy tissue. (Synonym: radiotherapy)

Radiology. The branch of medicine dealing with the use of x-rays and other forms of radiant energy in the diagnosis and treatment of disease. (Synonyms: x-ray, medical imaging)

Radiology department. That unit in a hospital specifically designed, equipped, and staffed to use x-rays and other radioactive elements for the diagnosis and treatment of patients. This department is under the direct supervision of a radiologist (physician). This department could also include radiation therapy and/or nuclear medicine sections. (Synonyms: x-ray department, medical imaging department)

Reasonable cost. Costs approved by third-party payers for reimbursement to a hospital, which are then included as a hospital's allowable costs determined by cost report. (Synonyms: cost reimbursement, total cost)

Rehabilitative medicine. Medical specialty concerned with the diagnosis and treatment of certain musculoskeletal defects and neuromuscular diseases including physical therapy, occupational therapy, speech therapy, and closely related specialties.

Residency. Any training following graduation from an approved medical college, which leads to certification in a specialty field of medicine. This training must be approved by the American Medical Association or the American Osteopathic Association.

Resident. A physician who has completed an internship or last year of medical school and is taking further supervised full-time hospital training in a specialty area of medicine. (Synonyms: house staff, postgraduate year [PGY])

Respiratory care department. An organizational unit of a hospital designed to provide ventilator support and associated services to patients. (Synonyms: respiratory therapy department, inhalation therapy department)

Risk management. The science of identifying, studying and controlling risks to patients, employees, and the hospital. An early warning system for identifying potential causes of liability.

Risk management committee. One of a hospital's quality improvement committees. The committee develops policies and procedures to enhance a safe environment, conducts surveillance programs to monitor all adverse occurrences, and reviews incidence reports.

Room and board. A hospital revenue category that includes revenue from room, board, and general nursing services. (Synonym: routine services or daily patient services; daily room and board)

School of nursing. A broad term used today as a catchall phrase for various forms of education offered to individuals pursuing a nursing career.

Security department. That unit or department of a hospital responsible for protecting patients, their families, and hospital staff as well as safeguarding the facility, equipment, and supplies.

Self pay. Individuals, institutions, or corporations assuming the entire responsibility for payment of hospital and medical bills that otherwise might be covered by an insurance policy. (Synonym: self-insured)

Semiprivate accommodations. Accommodations provided in a room of two or more beds (usually three or four) with a charge that would generally be less than private or single-bed accommodations.

Sentinel events. Unexpected hospital mishaps resulting in death or serious physical injury that must be reported to the JCAHO and investigated, seeking the root cause and instituting preventive changes.

Sexual harassment. Illegal activity prohibited either in the form of hostile work environment or quid pro quo (something for something). The EEOC is charged with investigation and if necessary, enforcement.

Shared purchasing. A co-op arrangement between hospitals to reduce the cost of purchases. (Synonym: group purchasing)

Skilled nursing facilities (SNF). Facilities providing long-term care to individuals requiring nursing care but not hospitalization. They include extended care facilities reimbursable by Medicare, as well as nursing homes reimbursable by Medicaid.

Social Security Administration (SSA). Founded in 1946. The bureau of the federal government that is responsible for the administration of Medicare, whose financing is under the direction of the Health Care Financing Administration (HCFA). The SSA is also responsible for administering a number of other programs including the Old Age Survivors and Disability Insurance Program.

Social service department. That hospital unit responsible for working with patients, their families, and the institution's professional staff to assist patients with personal, socioeconomic, and environmental problems related to their medical conditions.

Special diets. Foods or menus specially planned and prepared for individuals who need nutritional therapy to improve their overall health or to control disease. Such diets are usually prescribed for a patient by a physician. The type of special diets can include modifications in consistency (liquid, soft), or content (sodium or fat restricted, high/low calorie/protein, and diabetic).

Speech therapist. A professional, registered therapist who evaluates, diagnoses, and counsels individuals with communication disorders.

Stark 1. Statute prohibiting referral of patients to an entity that the physician or physician's family member has a monetary interest in.

Stark 2. Technical amendment modifying Stark 1 and creating certain safe harbors.

Student nurses. Individuals preparing for careers as licensed practical nurses (LPNs) or registered nurses (RNs). In addition to classroom studies, nursing students must complete many hours of hands-on clinical training in a variety of settings. They are closely supervised by both experienced nurses and instructors as they perform routine patient care activities. Nursing schools usually contract with hospitals, nursing homes, and other health care institutions to provide clinical training sites for their students.

Tax Equity and Fiscal Responsibility Act of 1982 (TEFRA). Public law 97-248, which covers many far-reaching Medicare amendments as applied to hospital reimbursement policies. This law was a first step in placing hospitals on a prospective pricing system (PPS) rather than the previous cost reimbursed, retrospective cost system.

Tax exempt revenue bonds. A source of debt financing for hospitals with two major features: the interest received by bondholders is not subject to federal income tax, and the organization receiving the financing secures the bonds with its gross revenues.

Teaching hospital. A hospital providing undergraduate or graduate medical education, usually with one or more medical or dental internships and/or residency programs in affiliation with a medical school.

Tertiary medicare care. Highly sophisticated diagnostic and therapeutic services given to patients with complex and serious medical conditions. This type of care is usually rendered at teaching hospitals or at university-affiliated hospitals.

Third-party payer. Any agency or organization that pays or insures a specific package of health or medical expenses on behalf of the beneficiaries or recipients. Examples include Blue Cross/Blue Shield plans, Medicare, Medicaid, and health maintenance organizations (HMOs).

Unit clerk. The individual who performs routine clerical or reception work on a nursing unit, including receiving patients and visitors, scheduling appointments, working with records, and assisting in communications.

Urgent admission. That patient requiring admission to the hospital for a clinical condition that would require admission for diagnosis and treatment within 48 hours; otherwise the patient's life or well being could be threatened. The other two categories for admission are emergency and elective.

Urgent care center. A freestanding facility providing minor emergency (not life-threatening) care, or basic health services on a nonscheduled basis. (Synonyms: urgicenter; "doc in the box," freestanding emergency department, walk-in clinic)

Utilization. A quantitative measure of the actual use of equipment, facilities, programs, services, and personnel. This measure can be a simple rate, such as the number of admissions per day for a particular unit, or the complex evaluation of an institution's efficiency in allocating its resources, known as utilization review (UR).

Utilization review (UR). The process of examining the appropriate need of a patient's hospital admission, services provided the patient's length of stay (LOS), and the hospital's discharge practices. This type of review is required by the JCAHO, Medicare, Medicaid, and many other third-party payers and regulatory agencies.

Utilization review committee. A committee of the medical staff or of the hospital composed of physicians, nurses, administrative representatives, and allied health personnel. The committee's function is to review inpatients' medical records and those of patients who have been discharged in order to determine the medical necessity for their treatment and hospital stay. This committee may also be involved in reviewing the discharge plans for hospitalized patients. This committee is one element in a hospital's quality improvement program.

Vice president/assistant administrator. An individual, holding an upper level management position in a hospital, responsible for certain discrete segments, units or functions within the hospital. This person reports directly to the hospital administrator, president/CEO, or the associate administrator.

Volunteer. An individual who works without financial compensation performing a variety of hospital tasks within various departments. Members of the hospital auxiliary are volunteers.

Volunteers, director of. That individual, frequently a department head, who organizes and directs the training and utilization of volunteers within a hospital. This includes recruiting, assigning, and coordinating volunteers in their work assignments, and maintaining records of volunteer hours worked and the types of services performed.

Workers' Compensation. Law found in all states, providing compensation to those injured on the job.

Appendix C

The Hospital: URLs

American Association of Colleges of Nursing — http://www.aacn.nche.edu

American College of Healthcare Executives — http://www.ache.org

American Health Lawyers Association — http://www.healthlawyers.org

American Hospital Association — http://www.aha.org

American Medical Association — http://www.ama-assn.org

American Nurses Association — http://www.nursingworld.org

American Osteopathic Association — http://www.osteopathic.org

Bioethics.net — http://www.bioethics.net

Centers for Disease Control and Prevention — http://www.cdc.gov

Centers for Medicare and Medicaid Services — http://www.cms.hhs.gov

Department of Health and Human Services — http://www.hhs.gov

Families USA — http://www.familiesusa.org

Healthcare Financial Management Association — http://www.hfma.org

Healthcare Financing Administration — http://www.hcfa.gov

Healthcare Law Net — http://www.healthcarelawnet.com

HIPAA — http://www.hipaa.org

Institute for Safe Medication Practices — http://www.ismp.org

Joint Commission on Accreditation of Healthcare Organizations	http://www.jcaho.org
Leapfrog	http://www.leapfroggroup.org
Medical Group Management Association	http://www.mgma.com
National Center for Health Statistics	http://www.cdc.gov/nchs
National Institute of Health	http://www.nih.gov
National Library of Medicine	http://www.nlm.nih.gov
Statistical Abstracts of the United States	http://www.census.gov/statab/www
WebMD	http://www.webmd.com

Index

A

ABC analysis (inventory), 148
abstracting medical records, 183
access to care comparisons, 244
accident room. *See* emergency department
accidents, avoiding. *See* safety
accountability. *See* authority; responsibility
accountants, 172
accounting, 172–173
accounts, patient, 174 175
accreditation, 190, 199–200, 207–212
   certification for physicians, 69
accrual accounting, 173
ACHE (American College of Health Care Executives),
   37
active staff, 72
ADA (Americans with Disabilities Act), 152
administrative support services, 145–155
   accreditation and, 209
   case studies, 253
   human resources department, 148–154
   materials management, 145–148
   telecommunications management, 155
   volunteer organizations, 154
administrative work, by nurses, 80–81
administrators, hospital. *See* CEOs; COOs
admissions
   admitting department, 59–63
   decline in, 11
   emergency department, 54–55, 61, 238
advanced directives, 203
adverse drug reactions, 198
advertising, 220–221
AHA (American Hospital Association), 213
alcohol testing, 153
alliances, 27
allied health personnel, 74–75

almshouses, 4–5
ALOS (average length of stay), 11
AMA (American Medical Association), 70
ambulance services, 239
American Association of Medical Social Workers, 126
American College of Health Care Executives (ACHE),
   37
American Dietetic Association, 121–122
American Hospital Association (AHA), 213
American Manual for Hospitals (AMH), 209
American Nurses Association (ANA), 78 79
Americans with Disabilities Act (ADA), 152
AMH (American Manual for Hospitals), 209
ANA (American Nurses Association), 78 79
ancillary services, 95–117
   anesthesiology department, 105–107
   cardiac care, 111–112
   clinical laboratory, 96–100
   imaging department, 100–103
   rehabilitative medicine, 112–113
   respiratory care, 109–110
anesthesiology department, 105–107
angiography, 103
annual reports, 220
appointment of governing body, 29
appointment of medical staff, 68, 70
   reappointment reviews, 73
appraisal of employee performance, 151
assigning beds, 63
assistant administrators. *See* COOs
associate staff, 72
Association of Patient Service Representatives, 129
attending staff, 72
audit committee, 73
audits, market, 222–224
audits, medical, 190–191
audits, physician, 223

authority. *See also* responsibility
   power relationships, 26
   pyramid organization, 22
   trustees. *See* trustees
automated quality improvement, 191–192
automatic clinical records, 182
autonomy, 202
auxiliaries (volunteer organizations), 154–155
auxiliary nursing personnel, 80
average length of stay (ALOS), 11

B

babies, care units for, 85
background checks, employee, 153
balance sheets, 166
barbiturates, control of, 115–116
bed assignments, 63
beds, number of, 9, 11, 239
   laundry services, 133–134
   patient care units, 81
bedside terminals, 91
beneficence, 203
benefits, employee, 151
bids for sales, 146
bill for services. *See* patient costs
billing, 174–175
bioethics, 201–205
biomedical engineering, 141–142
blood banking, 97
Blue Cross/Blue Shield, 162–163
board certification for physicians, 69
board of trustees, 26, 29–35
   functions of, 31–33
   quality improvement responsibilities, 191
boiler room section, 136
Bond, Thomas, 5
bonds, 169
booklets for patients, 60, 219
brand name drugs, 116
branding, 222
brochures, distributing, 60, 219–220
budgeting, 165–169
bulk food delivery system, 123
bureaucratic organizations, 21
business functions, 171–175
bylaws, 34–35, 73

C

Cabot, Richard C., 126
cafeteria services, 124
CAP (College of American Pathologists), 99–100
capital budgets, 165, 169

capital formation, 169
capitation, 160–161
cardiac patients, care for, 85, 111–112
care quality. *See* quality and quality improvement
case nursing, 86
case studies, 247–267
cash flow budgets, 165
CAT and CT scans, 101–102. *See also* imaging
   department
categorizations. *See* classifications and categories
catering services, 125
Catholic hospitals, 5
CCUs (coronary care units), 85
centralized purchasing, 146
centralized tray service, 123
CEOs (chief executive officers), 24, 37–42
   functions and activities of, 38–41
   planning responsibilities, 228–229
   selection and evaluation of, 33
certificates of accreditation. *See* accreditation
certificates of need (CONs), 231
certification for physicians, 69
CFOs (chief financial officers), 39, 171–172
chain of command, 22 23
chaplains, 128
charges to patient. *See* patient costs
chart of accounts, 172
chief executive officers (CEOs), 24, 37–42
   functions and activities of, 38–41
   planning responsibilities, 228–229
   selection and evaluation of, 33
chief financial officers (CFOs), 39, 171–172
chief operating officers (COOs), 24, 38–42
chief residents, 68–69
cineradiography, 101
claim management, 175
classifications and categories
   admissions, 61
   budgets, 165
   disasters, 140–141
   emergency services, 52–53
   hospital beds, 239
   hospitals, 9
   labor units, 154
   medical staff, 72
   nursing care delivery, 86–88
cleanliness of hospital. *See* environmental services
clerical functions, 80–81
clinical engineering. *See* biomedical engineering
clinical laboratory department, 96–100
clinical outcomes, measuring, 190, 191
clinical testing for preadmission, 61–62
closed staffs, 71–73
CME (continuing medical education), 69

coding medical records, 183
collection agencies, 175
collective spirit, 31
College of American Pathologists (CAP), 99–100
committees
  medical records, 184
  medical staff, 73
  morbidity and mortality, 189
  pharmacy and therapeutics, 114
  quality control mechanisms, 189
  trustees, 34–35
communication needs (case study), 261
community element (medical care system), 240–241
community hospitals, 9–10
  public relations, 219
competitive bidding for sales contracts, 146
computer-aided scheduling, 90
computerized preventive maintenance programs, 135
conduct restrictions, 75
CONs (certificates of need), 231
consent forms, 62–63, 202
  anesthesiology, 106
construction, financing, 169
consulting staff, 72
continuing medical education (CME), 69
contract management, 41, 142. *See also* outside
  contractors
contraindications, 197
convenience food system, 123
conventional food system, 123
cook–chill food system, 123
cook–freeze food system, 123
cooperative purchasing, 146
COOs (chief operating officers), 24, 38–42
CORFs (comprehensive outpatient rehabilitation
  facilities), 113
coronary care units (CCUs), 85
corporate branding, 222
corporate compliance programs, 175
corporate restructuring, 26
Cortez, Hernando, 4
cost of care comparisons, 244
cost reimbursement, 160
costs to hospitals. *See* expenses, hospital
costs to patients. *See* patient costs
Council of Nicaea, 4
courtesy staff, 72
CPA firms, 174
credentials committee, 73, 189
criminal background checks, 153
CRNAs (certified registered nurse anesthetists),
  105
CT and CAT scans. *See also* imaging department
cyclical scheduling, 90

D

Darling v. Charleston Community Memorial Hospital,
  33–34, 191
decentralized tray service, 123
defensive medicine, 195
delinquent patient accounts, 175
DePaul Hospital (St. Louis), 5
diagnostic related groups (DRGs), 7, 160
  assigning, 183
dialysis centers, 86
dietary department, 121–126
director of nurses (DON), 80
directors. *See* trustees
disaster planning, 139–141, 250
discharge planning, 127–128
dispending medications, 115
dispensaries, 6
distribution of medications, 115
division of labor, 22
"do no harm", 203
DON (director of nurses), 80
DRGs (diagnostic related groups), 7, 160
  assigning, 183
drugs (medications)
  employee screening, 153
  errors with, 197–198
  pharmacy, 113–117, 189
  preparation rooms, 83

E

EAPs (employee assistance programs), 151
early American hospitals, 4–6
ED (emergency department), 51–58, 238
education, 240
  dieticians, 121–122
  nursing, 78–79
  physician, 68–69
  social workers, 126
EEG (electroencephalography) testing, 110
EEOC (Equal Employment Opportunity Act),
  152, 256
EKG (electrocardiography) testing, 111–112
elective admissions, 61
electrocardiography testing, 111–112
electroencephalography testing, 110
electronic medical records, 181–182
emergency admissions, 61, 238
emergency department, 51–58, 238
emergency preparedness, 139–141, 250
employee assistance programs (EAPs), 151
employee information handbooks, 219
employment. *See* labor and staffing

Employment Retirement Income Security Act (ERISA), 152

EMTALA (Emergency Medical Treatment and Active Labor Act), 55, 58, 238

endowment fund, 173

enrichment, job, 150

environmental services, 131–133
  accreditation and, 209

EOQ (economic order quantity), 148

Equal Employment Opportunity Act (EEOC), 152

Equal Pay Act of 1963, 152

equipment
  financing, 169
  maintenance of, 142
  safety equipment, 139

ER. See emergency department

ERISA (Employment Retirement Income Security Act), 152

errors, medical, 197–200
  sentinel events, 211

ether, discovery of, 5–6, 105

ethics, 201–205

European operating room, 199

evacuations, 140

evaluation of hospitals. See accreditation; JCAHO

exchange cart system, 147

executive committee, 34, 73

executive vice presidents. See COOs (chief operating officers)

expanded food service programs, 126

expenses, hospital, 12–16
  advertising, 221
  cost of care in United States, 244
  defensive medicine, 195
  emergency department, 57
  food services, 123
  nursing services, 88

external disasters, types of, 140–141

external public, 219

F

facilities support service, 131–142

facility planning, 230–231

Fair Labor Standards Act (FLSA), 152

fairness, 203–204

fiduciary responsibility of trustees, 31–33

finances
  admitting department, role of, 60
  budgeting, 165–169
  business functions, 171–175
  cost of care in United States, 244
  discharge planning, 128
  emergency department, 57, 239

food services, 123

fundraising campaigns, 220, 225

generating revenue, 159–164

nursing services, 88

statements of, 166–169

fire safety, 139

Flexner, Abraham, 188

floating bonds, 169

FLSA (Fair Labor Standards Act), 152

fluoroscopy, 101

food services, 121–126

formal licensing, 212

formulary development, 114

Franklin, Benjamin, 5

freestanding imaging centers, 105

frozen ready food system, 123

functional nursing, 87

fund accounting, 172–173

fundraising campaigns, 220, 225

future
  CEOs, role of, 42
  health care, 42
  nursing shortage, 91–92
  operating rooms, 199
  quality improvement, 192

G

Gamma Knife technology, 103

general fund, 173

general safety, 137–139
  disaster planning, 139–141, 250
  parking facilities, 136
  of patient, 197–200
  privacy of patient information, 179–180
  waste removal, 132–133

generation of hospital power, 136

generic drugs, 116

goals and objectives, determining, 229

Gonzalez v. John J. Nork, 34

governing bodies. See trustees

government hospitals, 9

government involvement in hospitals, 240–241
  history of, 6–7

group purchasing, 146

H

hazardous waste removal, 132–133

health care quality. See quality and quality improvement

Health Care Quality Improvement Act, 75

health care trends, 9–12

health insurance, 162–163
  HIPAA legislation, 60, 152, 179–180
health insurance premiums, 13, 15–16
health maintenance organizations (HMOs), 160, 163
hierarchical organization, 22
Hill-Burton Act, 6–7
HIPAA (Health Insurance Portability and
  Accountability Act), 60, 152, 179–180
history
  accreditation and licensing, 207–213
  hospital planning, 227–228
  hospitals, numbers of, 3–7
  nursing services, 77–78
  quality improvement, 188
HMOs (health maintenance organizations), 160, 163
hospital administrators. *See* CEOs
hospital classifications, 9
hospital maintenance services, 134–136
hospital policies, 32
  avoiding medical errors, 198–199
  safety, 138–139
hospital staff. *See* labor and staffing
Hospital Standardization Program, 207
hospital support services, 119
  accreditation and, 209
  administrative support services, 145–155
    accreditation and, 209
    case studies, 253
    human resources department, 148–154
    materials management, 145–148
    telecommunications management, 155
    volunteer organizations, 154
  facilities support service departments, 131–142
  food services, 121–126
  pastoral care services, 128
  patient representatives, 129
  patient transportation services, 128–129
  social services, 126–128
Hospital Survey and Construction Act, 6–7
hospital systems, 12
  governing bodies, 33
hospital (word), origin of, 3
hospitalists, 74
hospitals, history of, 3–7
hospitals, numbers of, 11–12
Hôtel-Dieu (Paris), 4
housekeeping. *See* environmental services
human resources department, 148–154

I

ICUs (intensive care units), 85
imaging department, 100–105
infection control committee, 189

infectious waste removal, 132–133
information booklets, distributing. *See* patient information booklets
information systems, 173–174
  clinical laboratory, 99
inhalation therapy department. *See* respiratory care
  department
injuries, avoiding. *See* safety
inpatient element (medical care system), 238
inside activities, CEOs, 38–41
institutional branding, 222
institutional brochures, 60, 219–220
insurance claim submission, 175
intensive care units (ICUs), 85
internal disasters, types of, 140–141
internal public, 219
interviews for staff positions, 150
intoxicated patients in emergency departments, 58
inventory and inventory management, 147
issuing bonds, 169

J

JCAHO (Joint Commission on Accreditation of Health
  Care Organizations), 199–200, 207–212
JCI (Joint Commission International), 211
Jesus of Nazareth Hospital (Mexico City), 4
job analysis, 149
job descriptions, 149
job enrichment, 150
Joint Commission International (JCI), 211
Joint Commission on Accreditation of Health Care
  Organizations (JCAHO), 199–200, 207–212
justice, 203–204

K

Katrina, Hurricane, 139–140

L

labor and staffing, 148–154
  anesthesiology department, 107
  biomedical engineering, 142
  board of trustees. *See* trustees
  clinical laboratory, 98
  costs of, 13–14. *See also* expenses, hospital
  emergency department, 54–56
  employee information handbooks, 219
  environmental services, 132
  imaging department, 104
  line and staff functions, 23
  medical social workers, 126–128
  medical staff, 67–75. *See also* physicians

allied health personnel, 74–75
anesthesiologists, 106
hospitalists, 74
medical errors, 197–200, 211
overseas opportunities, 245
pharmacists and pharmacy technicians, 114
physical therapy, 112–113
planning responsibilities, 229
primary care physicians, 237
social workers, 126–128
nursing services, 77–92
medical errors, 198–199
shortage of nurses, 91–92
SNFs (skilled nursing facilities), 240
staffing and scheduling, 88–90
overseas opportunities, 245
pharmacy, 114
planning responsibilities, 228–230
shift scheduling. *See* scheduling
specialization, 22
Labor-Management Relations Act, 154
labor unions, 154, 240
laundry services, 133–134
leasing, 147
legal concerns
closed medical staffs, 72
consent forms, 62–63, 202
anesthesiology, 106
corporate compliance programs, 175
emergency department, 58
HIPAA legislation, 60, 152, 179–180
human resources, 152–153
medical malpractice, 194–196
medical records, 185. *See also* HIPAA
nonphysician staff, 75
physician restrictions, 75
liability. *See* legal concerns
licensing, 78, 152, 154, 207–208, 211–212
line functions, 23
linens, 133–134
location. *See* physical facilities
logs of patients (emergency department), 56
Long, Crawford, 5
long-range plans, 228, 230
long-term care facilities, 86
lounge (nursing unit), 83
LPNs (license practical nurses), 78
LVNs (licensed vocational nurses), 78

M

MacEachern, Malcolm, 126
magnetic resonance imagine (MRI), 101–102. *See also*
imaging department
maintenance department, 134–136

maintenance of equipment, 142
major external disasters, 141
malpractice, 194–196
managed care systems, 163
management
nurse managers, 80
organization charts, 24–25
pyramid organization, 22
relocated management team (case study), 266
of risk, 189, 193–196
span of control, 21
management information systems (MIS), 173–174
manual medical records, 181
market audits and analyses, 222–224, 229
market research, 222
market studies, 222–223
marketing, 217–225
mass media and press relations, 220
materials management, 145–148
meal services, 121–126
medical audits, 190–191
medical care quality. *See* quality and quality
improvement
medical committees. *See* committees
medical director, 74
medical errors, 197–200
sentinel events, 211
medical executive committee, 73
medical imaging department, 100–105
medical insurance, 162–163
HIPAA legislation, 60, 152, 179–180
medical malpractice, 194–196
medical outcomes, measuring, 190, 191
medical records, 179–185, 195. *See also* record
keeping
medical records department, 182–185
medical social workers, 126–128
medical staff, 67–75. *See also* labor and staffing
allied health personnel, 74–75
anesthesiologists, 106
hospitalists, 74
medical errors, 197–200, 211
nursing services, 77–92
medical errors, 198–199
shortage of nurses, 91–92
SNFs (skilled nursing facilities), 240
staffing and scheduling, 88–90
overseas opportunities, 245
physical therapy, 112–113
physicians. *See* physicians
planning responsibilities, 229
primary care physicians, 237
medical technologists, 98, 104
Medicare and Medicaid legislation, 7, 13, 14, 113,
160–162, 212, 238

medications
  employee drug screening, 153
  errors with, 197–198
  pharmacy, 113–117, 189
  preparation rooms, 83
membership status, 72
mental hospitals, 5
menus, patient, 122
middle management, 24
minor external disasters, 141
minors as patients, in emergency rooms, 58
MIS (management information systems), 173–174
mobile imaging centers, 105
morbidity and mortality committee, 189
mortality rates, 244–245
Morton, William T. G., 5, 105
motivation, 150
MRI scans, 101–102. *See also* imaging department
multi-bed rooms, 81
multihospital systems, 12
  governing bodies, 33

N

name branding, 222
narcotics, control of, 115–116
National Practitioner Data Bank, 75
needles, discarded, 133
negligence, 194–196
negotiated bids, 160
negotiation of contracts. *See* contract management
neonatal intensive care units, 85
networked departments, 174
newsletters for hospitals, 219
NLN (National League for Nursing), 79
NLRB (National Labor Relations Board), 154
nonacute special care units, 85
nonmaleficence, 203
nonphysician staff, 74–75
nuclear medicine, 102, 112
nurse anesthetists, 105, 107
nurses' station, 81–82
nursing home care, 86
nursing services, 77–92
  medical errors, 198–199
  shortage of nurses, 91–92
  SNFs (skilled nursing facilities), 240
  staffing and scheduling, 88–90
nursing units. *See* patient care units

O

objectives and goals, determining, 229
Occupational Safety and Health Administration
  (OSHA), 137

occupational therapy, 112–113
off-label use of medications, 198
open staffs, 71–73
operating budgets, 165
operating room errors, 199
OR (operating room), errors in, 199
organization, 21–27
  accreditation and, 209
  anesthesiology department, 106
  CEOs. *See* CEOs
  charts of, 24–25
  clinical laboratory, 97
  emergency department, 54
  governing bodies. *See* trustees
  imaging department, 103
  medical records department, 183
  medical staff, 70
  nursing services, 80
  quality control mechanisms, 189
organizations, Web sites for, 299
organized medicine, 70
orientation programs for new staff, 150
ORYX initiative, 190
OSHA (Occupational Safety and Health
  Administration), 137
OT (occupational therapy), 112–113
outcomes, clinical, 190, 191
outpatient pharmacies, 114
outpatient procedures, 11, 17, 238
  CORFs (comprehensive outpatient rehabilitation
    facilities), 113
  imaging department, 103
outreach element (medical care system), 237
outside activities, CEOs, 38–41
outside contractors
  food services, 125
  liability for actions of, 195
  maintenance services, 135
  managing contracts, 41, 142
  planning advice, 228
  transcription services, 184
overseas opportunities, 245

P

parking facilities, 136–137
pastoral care services, 128
pathology departments. *See* clinical laboratory
  department
patient accounts and billing, 174–175
patient acuity systems, 89
patient autonomy, 203
patient care units, 80–83
patient costs
  cost of care in United States, 244

emergency department, 239
  pricing decisions, 223
patient information booklets, 60, 219
patient log (emergency department), 56
patient menus, 122
patient records. *See* record keeping
patient relations, CEO role in, 40
patient representatives, 129
patient safety. *See* safety
patient support services, 121–129
  food services, 121–126
  pastoral care services, 128
  patient representatives, 129
  social services, 126–128
  transportation services, 128–129
patient transportation services, 128–129
Patient's Bill of Rights, 60
payments. *See* revenues, hospital
payors, major, 161–164
peer review organizations (PROs), 189–190
Pennsylvania Hospital, 5
performance, employee, 151
permission slips. *See* consent forms
personnel. *See* labor and staffing
personnel department. *See* human resources
  department
PET (positron emission tomography), 102
Pete Marivich Center, 140
pharmacy, 113–117, 189
PHI (protected health information), 180
physiatrists, 112
physical facilities
  accreditation and, 209
  anesthesiology department, 106–107
  clinical laboratory, 98–99
  dietary department, 124
  emergency department, 53–54
  environmental services, 131–133, 209
  imaging department, 104
  laundry services, 133–134
  maintenance services, 134–136
  operating rooms, 199
  physical therapy, 113
  planning, 230–231
physical plant, 136
  accreditation and, 209
  funding, 173
physical safeguards for patient information, 180
physical therapy, 112–113
physicians, 68–69
  anesthesiologists, 106
  auditing, 223
  emergency department coverage, 55–56
  legal restrictions, 75

liability for actions of, 195
  medical errors, 197–200, 211
  occupational therapy, 113
  primary care (solo practitioners), 237
Pinel, Philippe, 5
planning, 227–231
  budgets, 165–169
  for disasters, 139–141, 250
  position control, 149
  for safety, 136
plant engineering, 136
  accreditation and, 209
plant fund, 173
policies, hospital, 32
  avoiding medical errors, 198–199
  safety, 138–139
Polygraph Protection Act, 153
position control plans, 149
positioning strategies, 223
power plant, 136
power relationships, 26
PPOs (preferred provider organizations), 160, 163
PR (public relations), 218–220
  admitting department, 59–60
  telecommunications management, 155
preadmission, 61–62
preferred provider organizations (PPOs), 160, 163
Pregnancy Discrimination Act, 153
premiums (health insurance), 13, 15–16
press relations and mass media, 220
preventive maintenance, 135
pricing, 223. *See also* patient costs
primary care nursing, 87–88
primary care physicians, 237
privacy of patient information, 179–180
private insurance, 163
private rooms (single-bed), 81
process audits, 191
professional conduct, 75
professional review organizations (PROs), 189–190
professional service departments. *See* ancillary services
profit-and-loss statements, 166
promotion, 223
PROs (peer review organizations), 189–190
prospective payment system (DRGs), 7, 160
  assigning, 183
protected health information (PHI), 180
provisional staff, 72
psychiatric social workers, 128
PT (physical therapy), 112–113
PTAs (physical therapy assistants), 113
public accounting firms, 174
public relations, 218–220
  admitting department, 59–60

telecommunications management, 155
public relations, CEO role in, 40
publications, 219
purchasing section (materials management), 146–147
pyramid organization, 22

Q

qualifications. *See* education
quality and quality improvement, 187–192
  accreditation and, 209
  appraisal of employee performance, 151
  avoiding medical errors, 198–199
  clinical laboratory, 99–100
  committee for quality improvement, 73
  Health Care Quality Improvement Act, 75
  medical records. *See also* HIPAA
  pharmacy, 117
  risk management and, 194
  social workers, 127–128
  US medical care system, 235–245

R

radiation therapy, 103
radiology. *See* imaging department
random drug screening, 153
ratio analysis, 166
reappointment reviews, 73
receiving section (materials management), 147
recertification practices, 69
record keeping, 56
  accounting, 172–173
  automatic clinical records, 91
  medical records, 179–185
  role of medical records, 195
recruitment, 150
references, job, 153
registered nurses (RNs), 87
registered technologists, 98, 104
registration, 212–213
rehabilitative medicine, 112–113
relationship management. *See* public relations
releasing medical records, 185
relicensing, nurses, 78
religious services for patients, 128
relocated management team (case study), 266
renal dialysis centers, 86
Renaudot, Théophraste, 6
renovation, 135–136, 169
residency programs, 68
respiratory care department, 109–110
respondent superior, 39, 195
responsibility. *See also* authority

CEOs, 38–41
teams, 23
  JCAHO survey teams, 209–210
  relocated management team (case study), 266
  risk management, 193
  of three, 26
  of trustees, 29–33
revenues, hospital, 12–13, 159–164
  ancillary services, 95
  emergency department, 57
  fundraising campaigns, 220, 225
  statements of, 166
risk management, 189, 193–196
RNs (registered nurses), 87
rooms, patient, 81
root cause analyses, 211
rotating coverage, 55
rules systems, 21
  bylaws, 34–35, 73
rural hospitals, 12

S

safeguards for patient information, 180
safety, 137–139
  disaster planning, 139–141, 250
  parking facilities, 136
  of patient, 197–200
  privacy of patient information, 179–180
  waste removal, 132–133
salary and wages, 151
  trustees, 30
sale of drugs to hospitals, 116
sales functions, 221–222
sanitary specialists. *See* environmental services
scheduling
  interviews for staff positions, 150
  nursing staff, 89–90
  parking needs, 136
  patient menus, 122
  preadmission and, 62
schooling. *See* education
security, 137
  disaster planning, 139–141, 250
security of drugs, 115–117
self-governance, 40
self-paying patients, 163–164
semiprivate patient rooms, 81
sentinel events, 211
sexual harassment, 153, 256
shared purchasing, 146
shift scheduling. *See* scheduling
shortage of nurses, 91–92
single-bed (private) rooms, 81

skilled nursing facilities (SNFs), 240
SNFs (skilled nursing facilities), 240
social justice, 203–204
social services department, 126–128
solo practitioners, 237
span of control, 21
special care units, 83–86
special diets for hospital patients, 122–123
special fund, 173
specialization of labor, 22
specialty boards and associations, 68
specific services method of payment, 160
SPECT (single photon emission computed
    tomography), 103
speech therapy, 112–113
staffing. See labor and staffing
standards of nursing care, 88
statistical analysis of patient records, 183
statistical reports, 166–169
stereoscopy, 101
storage of inventory, 147
strategic planning, 229–230
structure audits, 190
subterranean parking, 136–137
suing the hospital, 194–195
support services, 119
    accreditation and, 209
    administrative support services, 145–155
        accreditation and, 209
        case studies, 253
        human resources department, 148–154
        materials management, 145–148
        telecommunications management, 155
        volunteer organizations, 154
    facilities support service departments, 131–142
    food services, 121–126
    pastoral care services, 128
    patient representatives, 129
    patient transportation services, 128–129
    social services, 126–128
surface parking, 136–137
surgical errors, 199
survey, JCAHO, 209–210
SWOT analysis, 229
systems of hospitals. See hospital systems
systems of rules, 21
    bylaws, 34–35, 73

T

Taft-Hartley Act, 154
target markets, 221
tax-exempt revenue bonds, 169
team nursing, 87

teams, 23
    JCAHO survey teams, 209–210
    relocated management team (case study), 266
    risk management, 193
    of three, 26
technical safeguards for patient information, 180
technicians (technologists), 98, 104
telecommunications management, 155
telemonitoring, 91
temporary staff, 72
testing for preadmission, 61–62
therapeutics committee, 114, 189
therapists. See medical staff
third-party payments, 159–161
tissue committee, 73, 97
    quality control, 189
tort law, 194–195
towel (case study), 249
traditional scheduling of nursing staff, 89–90
training. See education
transcription of medical records, 184
transplantations, 6
transportation services (for patients), 128–129
trauma centers, 52
tray service (food), 123
trends
    CEOs, role of, 42
    electronic medical records, 181–182
    management information systems (MIS), 174
    nursing shortage, 91–92
    quality improvement, 192
triple A nurses, 88
troubled employees, dealing with, 151
trustees, 26, 29–35
    functions of, 31–33
    quality improvement responsibilities, 191

U

ultrasound imaging, 102
uninsured patients, 13
unions, 154, 240
unit clerks, 80–81
urban hospitals, 12
URLs, list of, 299
US medical care system, 235–241
    compared to the world, 243–245
utility room (nursing units), 83
utilization review (UR), 188, 189

V

van Heerden, Ivor, 140
vending services, 124–125

vice president of nursing. *See* director of nurses (DON)
vice presidents. *See* COOs (chief operating officers)
vision statements, 229
voluntary coverage, 55
volunteer organizations, 154–155

W

wages and salary, 151
  trustees, 30
ward clerks, 80–81

warehousing, 147
waste removal, 132–133
Web sites for hospitals, 219, 222
Web sites for organizations, list of, 299
wheelchair services, 129
work orders, 135
worker's compensation, 153

X

x-rays. *See* imaging department